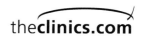

ORAL AND MAXILLOFACIAL SURGERY CLINICS
of North America

Management of Impacted Teeth

VINCENT J. PERCIACCANTE, DDS
Guest Editor

RICHARD H. HAUG, DDS
Consulting Editor

February 2007 • Volume 19 • Number 1

SAUNDERS

An Imprint of Elsevier, Inc.
PHILADELPHIA   LONDON   TORONTO   MONTREAL   SYDNEY   TOKYO

W.B. SAUNDERS COMPANY

A Division of Elsevier Inc.

1600 John F. Kennedy Blvd., Suite 1800, Philadelphia, PA 19103-2899

http://www.oralmaxsurgery.theclinics.com

ORAL AND MAXILLOFACIAL SURGERY	**Volume 19, Number 1**
CLINICS OF NORTH AMERICA	**ISSN 1042-3699**
February 2007	**ISBN-13: 978-1-4160-4345-4**
Editor: John Vassallo; j.vassallo@elsevier.com	**ISBN-10: 1-4160-4345-4**

Reprints. For copies of 100 or more, of articles in this publication, please contact the Commercial Reprints Department, Elsevier Inc., 360 Park Avenue South, New York, New York 10010-1710. Tel. (212) 633-3813; Fax: (212) 462-1935; e-mail: reprints@elsevier.com.

The ideas and opinions expressed in *Oral and Maxillofacial Surgery Clinics of North America* do not necessarily reflect those of the Publisher. The Publisher does not assume any responsibility for any injury and/or damage to persons or property arising out of or related to any use of the material contained in this periodical. The reader is advised to check the appropriate medical literature and the product information currently provided by the manufacturer of each drug to be administered to verify the dosage, the method and duration of administration, or contraindications. It is the responsibility of the treating physician or other health care professional, relying on independent experience and knowledge of the patient, to determine drug dosages and the best treatment for the patient. Mention of any product in this issue should not be construed as endorsement by the contributors, editors, or the Publisher of the product or manufacturers' claims.

Oral and Maxillofacial Surgery Clinics of North America (ISSN 1042-3699) is published quarterly by Elsevier Inc., 360 Park Avenue South, New York, NY 10010-1710. Months of issue are February, May, August, and November. Business and Editorial Offices: 1600 John F. Kennedy Blvd., Suite 1800, Philadelphia, PA 19103-2899. Customer Service Office: 6277 Sea Harbor Drive, Orlando, FL 32887-4800. Periodicals postage paid at New York, NY and additional mailing offices. Subscription prices are $218.00 per year for US individuals, $325.00 per year for US institutions, $101.00 per year for US students and residents, $252.00 per year for Canadian individuals, $380.00 per year for Canadian institutions, $274.00 per year for international individuals, $380.00 per year for international institutions and $129.00 per year for Canadian and foreign students/residents. To receive student/resident rate, orders must be accompanied by name or affiliated institution, date of term, and the *signature* of program/residency coordinator on institution letterhead. Orders will be billed at individual rate until proof of status is received. Foreign air speed delivery is included in all *Clinics* subscription prices. All prices are subject to change without notice. **POSTMASTER:** Send address changes to *Oral and Maxillofacial Surgery Clinics of North America*, Elsevier Periodicals Customer Service, 6277 Sea Harbor Drive, Orlando, FL 32887-4800. **Customer Service: 1-800-654-2452 (US). From outside of the US, call 1-407-345-4000**.

Printed in the United States of America.

GUEST EDITOR

VINCENT J. PERCIACCANTE, DDS, Assistant Professor and Residency Program Director, Division of Oral and Maxillofacial Surgery, Emory University School of Medicine, Atlanta, Georgia

CONTRIBUTORS

PAMELA L. ALBERTO, DMD, Clinical Associate Professor and Director of Predoctoral Surgery, Department of Oral and Maxillofacial Surgery, University of Medicine and Dentistry of New Jersey, New Jersey Dental School, Newark, New Jersey

JOHN M. ALLEN, DMD, Former Attending Staff, Division of Oral and Maxillofacial Surgery, Emory University School of Medicine, Atlanta, Georgia

SHAHROKH C. BAGHERI, DMD, MD Clinical Assistant Professor, Division of Oral and Maxillofacial Surgery, Emory University; Private Practice, Atlanta Oral and Facial Surgery, Atlanta, Georgia

JEFFREY BENNETT, DMD, Professor and Chair, Department of Oral Surgery and Hospital Dentistry, Indiana University School of Dentistry, Indianapolis, Indiana

GARY F. BOULOUX, MD, BDS, MDSc, FRACDS, FRACDS(OMS), Assistant Professor, Division of Oral and Maxillofacial Surgery, Emory University School of Medicine, Atlanta, Georgia

THOMAS B. DODSON, DMD, MPH, Associate Professor and Visiting Oral and Maxillofacial Surgeon, and Director, Center of Applied Clinical Investigation, Departments of Oral and Maxillofacial Surgery, Harvard School of Dental Medicine, Massachusetts General Hospital, Boston, Massachusetts

SAM E. FARISH, DMD, Chief, Division of Oral and Maxillofacial Surgery, Atlanta Veterans Affairs Medical Center; and Assistant Professor, Division of Oral and Maxillofacial Surgery, Emory University School of Medicine, Atlanta, Georgia

JAMES R. HUPP, DMD, MD, JD, MBA, Dean, School of Dentistry and Professor, Department of Oral and Maxillofacial Surgery, University of Mississippi Medical Center, Jackson, Mississippi

HUSAIN ALI KHAN, DMD, MD, Private Practice, Atlanta Oral and Facial Surgery, Atlanta, Georgia

ROBERT D. MARCIANI, DMD, Professor of Surgery and Chief, Division of Oral and Maxillofacial Surgery, University of Cincinnati, Ohio

MEHRAN MEHRABI, DMD, MD, Former Resident, Division of Oral and Maxillofacial Surgery, Emory University School of Medicine, Atlanta, Georgia

VINCENT J. PERCIACCANTE, DDS, Assistant Professor and Residency Program Director, Division of Oral and Maxillofacial Surgery, Emory University School of Medicine, Atlanta, Georgia

M. ANTHONY POGREL, DDS, MD, FRCS, FACS, Professor and Chairman, Department of Oral and Maxillofacial Surgery, University of California, San Francisco, California

DANIEL T. RICHARDSON, DMD, MD, Oral and Maxillofacial Surgery Resident-in-Training, Departments of Oral and Maxillofacial Surgery, Harvard School of Dental Medicine, Massachusetts General Hospital, Boston, Massachusetts

STEVEN M. ROSER, DMD, MD, Professor and Chief, Division of Oral and Maxillofacial Surgery, Emory University School of Medicine, Atlanta, Georgia

MARTIN B. STEED, DDS, Division of Oral and Maxillofacial Surgery, Emory University School of Medicine, Atlanta, Georgia

TREVOR TREASURE, DDS, MD, MBA, Assistant Professor and Program Director, Oral and Maxillofacial Surgery Residency, Indiana University School of Dentistry, Indianapolis, Indiana

VINCENT B. ZICCARDI, DDS, MD, Associate Professor and Chair, Department of Oral and Maxillofacial Surgery, University of Medicine and Dentistry of New Jersey, Newark, New Jersey

JOHN R. ZUNIGA, DMD, MS, PhD, Professor and Chair, Division of Oral and Maxillofacial Surgery, University of Texas Medical Center, Dallas, Texas

CONTENTS

Asymptomatic third molars may have associated periodontal pathology that may not be limited to the third molar region and have a negative impact on systemic health. Third molars should be considered for removal when there is clinical, radiographic, or laboratory evidence of acute or chronic periodontitis, caries, pericoronitis, deleterious effects on second molars, or pathology. Radiographic findings of extreme locations of impacted teeth, dense bone, dilacerated roots, large radiolucent lesions associated with impactions, and lower third molar apices in cortical inferior border bone are predictive of more complex surgery. Certain demographic and oral health conditions available to the surgeon before surgery and intraoperative circumstances are predictive of delayed recovery for health-related quality of outcomes and delayed clinical outcomes after third molar surgery.

Surgical removal of impacted third molars is the most commonly performed procedure by oral and maxillofacial surgeons. The removal of diseased or symptomatic third molars has not been an issue of controversy. The risk of surgery and associated complications are justified and uniformly accepted by most surgeons when the teeth are associated with chronic or acute pathologic processes, including caries, nonrestorable teeth, fractured roots, resorption, associated pathologic conditions (cysts, tumors), periapical abscesses, odontogenic infections, osteomyelitis, removal before reconstructive or ablative surgery, and radiation therapy.

The most commonly performed surgical procedure in most oral and maxillofacial surgery practices is the removal of impacted third molars. Extensive training, skill, and experience allow this procedure to be performed in an atraumatic fashion with local anesthesia, sedation, or general anesthesia. The decision to remove symptomatic third molars is not usually difficult, but the decision to remove asymptomatic third molars is sometimes less clear and requires clinical experience. A wide body of literature (discussed elsewhere in this issue) attempts to establish clinical practice guidelines for dealing with impacted teeth. Data is beginning to accumulate from third molar studies, which hopefully will provide surgeons and their patients with evidence-based guidelines regarding elective third molar surgery.

an intimate relationship between the roots of the mandibular third molar and the inferior alveolar nerve.

Risk of Periodontal Defects After Third Molar Surgery: An Exercise in Evidence-based Clinical Decision-making
Thomas B. Dodson and Daniel T. Richardson

This article's purpose is to apply evidence-based principles to answer the question: What is the risk of having persistent or new periodontal defects on the distal aspect of the mandibular second molar after third molar removal? Commonly, the second molar periodontal health either remains unchanged or improves after third molar removal. Eighteen weeks or more after third molar removal, 52% to 100% of subjects had no change or improvement in attachment levels or probing depths. For subjects with healthy second molar periodontium preoperatively, the indication for third molar removal should be evaluated carefully because these patients have an increased risk for worsening of probing depths or attachment levels after third molar removal.

Is There a Role for Reconstructive Techniques to Prevent Periodontal Defects After Third Molar Surgery?
Thomas B. Dodson

The purpose of this article is to address the following clinical question: Among subjects undergoing mandibular third molar (M3) removal, does an intervention at the time of tooth removal, when compared with no intervention, improve the long-term periodontal health on the distal aspect of the adjacent second molar (M2)? Routine application of interventions to improve the periodontal parameters on the distal of the M2 at the time of M3 removal is not indicated for most subjects. There seems to be a subpopulation of subjects having M3s removed who are at increased risk for periodontal defects after M3 removal, pre-existing periodontal defects, and a horizontal or mesioangular impaction. In the clinical setting of all three risk factors being present, there seems to be a predictable benefit to treating the dentoalveolar defect at the time of extraction.

Nerve Injuries After Third Molar Removal
Vincent B. Ziccardi and John R. Zuniga

Trigeminal nerve injuries are a known complication of third molar surgery. This article reviews the diagnosis, assessment, classification, microsurgical management, and outcome assessment of trigeminal nerve injuries that result from third molar removal.

Complications of Third Molar Surgery
Gary F. Bouloux, Martin B. Steed, and Vincent J. Perciaccante

This article addresses the incidence of specific complications and, where possible, offers a preventive or management strategy. Injuries of the inferior alveolar and lingual nerves are significant issues that are discussed separately in this text. Surgical removal of third molars is often associated with postoperative pain, swelling, and trismus. Factors thought to influence the incidence of complications after third molar removal include age, gender, medical history, oral contraceptives, presence of pericoronitis, poor oral hygiene, smoking, type of impaction, relationship of third molar to the inferior alveolar nerve, surgical time, surgical technique, surgeon experience, use of perioperative antibiotics, use of topical antiseptics, use of intra-socket medications, and anesthetic technique. Complications that are discussed further include alveolar osteitis, postoperative infection, hemorrhage, oro-antral communication, damage to adjacent teeth, displaced teeth, and fractures.

FORTHCOMING ISSUES

PREVIOUS ISSUES

ELSEVIER
SAUNDERS

Oral Maxillofacial Surg Clin N Am 19 (2007) xi

**ORAL AND
MAXILLOFACIAL
SURGERY CLINICS**
of North America

Preface

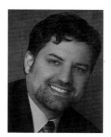

Vincent J. Perciaccante, DDS
Guest Editor

When Richard Haug presented to me the opportunity to be a Guest Editor for the *Oral and Maxillofacial Surgery Clinics of North America*, he gave me latitude in the topics that the volume would cover. My initial considerations went to orthognathic surgery, facial aesthetic surgery, and trauma, because these are my three biggest areas of interest. As part of the decision-making process, I reviewed the topics that were covered in the *Clinics* in the past and their timing to determine what would be the most pertinent and useful. The more I thought about it, I came to the realization that a topic that deserved attention—one that is most pertinent to all oral and maxillofacial surgeons—and is a part of our specialty that I enjoy is the *management of impacted teeth.*

Oral and maxillofacial surgeons are involved with the management of impacted teeth nearly every working day during their career. With the ongoing third molar studies supported by the American Association of Oral and Maxillofacial Surgeons and the Oral and Maxillofacial Surgery Foundation, more evidence-based information is coming to light on this topic, which will have an impact on our decisions and practices. If we neglect to continue in the trend of systematic evaluation of this subject, we risk trivializing one of the most commonly performed surgical procedures. Continued research and reinforcement of its value in practice and teaching are important for the care of our patients.

I was extremely pleased by the interest and willingness of the contributors to write on this subject. We have tried to cover the topic from all aspects: the decision to treat, techniques, interventions, and therapeutics, avoidance and management of complications, and management of risk.

I have truly enjoyed the experience of participating in the process of publishing this work, and I hope you find this issue useful. I would like to thank my wife, Amy, and my family for their continued support in my career, and my mentors, Bob Bays, Tom Dodson, Sam Farish, and Steve Roser, for their guidance.

Vincent J. Perciaccante, DDS
*Division of Oral and Maxillofacial Surgery
Emory University School of Medicine
1365-B Clifton Road NE
Suite 2300-B
Atlanta, GA 30322*

E-mail address: vpercia@emory.edu

ELSEVIER
SAUNDERS

Oral Maxillofacial Surg Clin N Am 19 (2007) 1–13

ORAL AND
MAXILLOFACIAL
SURGERY CLINICS
of North America

Third Molar Removal: An Overview of Indications, Imaging, Evaluation, and Assessment of Risk

Robert D. Marciani, DMD

*Division of Oral and Maxillofacial Surgery, University of Cincinnati, 231 Albert Sabin Way,
PO Box 670558, Cincinnati, OH 45267-0558, USA*

Surgical management of impacted third molars is a common treatment routinely dispensed in the private offices of oral and maxillofacial surgeons. Removing asymptomatic third molars is not without controversy and debate. Critics of this practice argue that in the absence of demonstrated disease, symptoms, or orthodontic considerations, patients are subjected to unnecessary pain, surgical risk, and adverse economic consequences [1–3]. "Consumers Report Medical Guide" identified "12 surgeries patients may be better off without." According to the "Consumer Reports Medical Guide," "third molar removal" is one health care treatment—along with hysterectomies and gastric bypasses—that the public might not need [4].

Health care economics, including the prudent and efficient distribution of resources society commits to health care and disability, continue to engender intense health policy disputes. Health policy debates by government and industry and the decisions that result from this activity heavily influence the distribution of medical and dental "goods and services." Oral and maxillofacial surgeons are responsible for making evidence-based health care decisions for the treatments they render to trusting patients. Third molar surgery is a segment of practice that has drawn considerable public attention and requires compelling evidence that "asymptomatic wisdom teeth" should by removed. Discussing the "indications, imaging, evaluation and assessment of risk" of third molar removal is only pertinent

after an argument is made for why asymptomatic third molars should be considered for removal.

Choosing a treatment option for patients should be guided by (1) establishing sound defensible diagnostic criteria that a condition exists and is amenable to treatment, (2) ensuring that the care rendered should be predictably effective with increasing levels of certainty the more elective the procedure, (3) making the patient aware of the consequences of treatment versus no treatment, (4) considering health-related quality-of-life (HQOL) issues along with clinical issues, and (5) considering the cost to society in the final decision for treatment.

Population studies in Sweden indicated that 80% of adolescent and young adults have four third molars and only 5% have no third molars [5]. Extrapolating the Swedish population's studies to similar cohorts in the United States suggests that almost every young adult must decide whether to have surgery to remove the third molars or retain and monitor the third molars until problems arise. Important health-related questions are best resolved when the diagnostic dilemma or the efficacy of a particular approach to management of an illness or a condition is studied prospectively under the most vigorous of scientific protocols. Until recently, few population-based studies have been conducted to determine the prevalence of pericoronitis. Few data exist to characterize over time the prevalence of periodontal defects on second molars or around retained third molars.

Blakey and colleagues [6] reported a higher prevalence of increased periodontal probing depths (PD) in the third molar region than clinicians expected. At baseline, 25% of the sample of 329 subjects enrolled in a longitudinal trial

E-mail address: marciard@ucmail.uc.edu

had at least 1 PD ≥ 5 mm in the third molar region; one third of subjects at least 25 years of age had at least 1 PD ≥ 5 mm. Only 4 subjects had PD $\geq$ anterior to the third molar region. White and colleagues [7] documented that the same subjects who had a PD ≥ 5 mm at baseline had elevated levels of "orange" and "red" complex periodontal pathogens detected in biofilm samples from the distal of second molars and elevated levels of gingival crevicular fluid mediators, interleukin-1β. The effects of a smoldering periodontal condition have health implications beyond the oral cavity. Chronic oral inflammation associated with periodontal disease has been implicated in increasing the risk for cardiovascular disease and renal insufficiency and preterm births [8–11]. Endothelial cell activation is the common cause for these clinical conditions in the oral cavity and at remote sites.

In a later study, Blakey and colleagues [12] assessed the changes in periodontal depth over time in the third molar region, the distal of second molars, or around third molars, as a clinical indication of worsening periodontal pathology in subjects retaining asymptomatic third molars. The data for these assessments were part of a study of subjects enrolled with four asymptomatic third molars with adjacent second molars in an institutional review board–approved longitudinal trial. Subjects were categorized as persons who exhibited a change ≥ 2 mm. Subjects with and without changes in PD were compared with Cochran-Mantel-Haenzsel statistics. Data from 254 subjects with a least two annual follow-up visits were available for analysis. Median follow-up from baseline to the second follow-up visit was 2.2 years. At enrollment, 59% of the subjects had at least 1 PD ≥ 4 mm in the third molar region, 25% had a PD ≥ 5 mm. Twenty-four percent of the subjects had at least one tooth that had an increased PD ≥ 2 mm in the third molar area at follow-up. Only 3% of those who had all teeth with a PD of <4 mm at baseline exhibited a change of ≥ 2 mm.

Blakey and his co-investigators' [12] latest study suggest that clinical findings of a PD ≥ 4 mm in the third molar region without symptoms may not be benign. White and colleagues [13] have reported that even in relatively young subjects (median age 28) increased PD is accompanied by high levels of periodontal pathogens and gingival crevicular fluid inflammatory mediators. A systemic response to the chronic oral inflammation might follow. Data obtained on 5831 persons

aged 18 to 34 from the Third National Health and Nutrition Examination Survey also showed an association between visible third molars and periodontal pathology in two randomly selected (one maxillary and one mandibular) quadrants [14]. Periodontal measures included gingival index, pocket depth, and attachment level on mesiobuccal and buccal sites on up to seven teeth (excluding third molars) per quadrant. Second molars were compared for periodontal pathology based on the presence or absence of a visible third molar in the same quadrant. A visible third molar was associated with twice the odds of a PD ≥ 5 mm on the adjacent second molar while controlling for other factors associated with visible third molars and periodontal disease. Other factors positively associated with PD ≥ 5 in the model were patient age of 25 to 34 years, smoking, and African American race.

In addition to the potential for periodontal problems associated with asymptomatic third molars, Shugars and colleagues [15] reported an association between caries experience in asymptomatic third molars and caries in restorations in first or second molars. In their cross-sectional analysis, one third of the study population had caries in third molars. Almost all of the patients with third molar caries experience had caries experience in a first or second molar. In contrast, the absence of caries experience in the first of second molars was associated with caries-free third molars. In a later study, Shugars and colleagues [16] investigated the incidence of occlusal caries in asymptomatic retained third molars erupted to the occlusal plane and examined the association between caries experience in other molars at baseline and incidence of caries experience in third molars over time. Their findings from this longitudinal analysis, coupled with the increased emphasis on a patient's cumulative caries experience as a predictor of future caries, suggest that more than 40% of patients aged 25 years old or older can expect caries experience in a third molar before the end of the third decade of life. Mandibular molars seem more susceptible than maxillary molars. Shugars and colleagues opined that patients in their third decade with vertically positioned noncarious third molars at the occlusal plane with good periodontal support and first and second molars with no caries experience are at low risk for caries development unless the patient's overall health status deteriorates. In a patient who has caries experience in first or second molars and who is just completing skeletal growth

Box 2. Patient factors predicting increased difficulty of third molar removal

Obesity
Dense bone
Large tongue
Dilacerated roots
Strong gag reflex
Position of the inferior alvelolar canal
Advanced age
Superiorly positioned maxillary third
  molar
Fractious patient
Apical root of lower third molar in
  cortical bone
Uneven anesthetic
Atrophic mandible
Limited surgical access
Location of maxillary sinus

additional imaging to prevent altered lower lip sensation.

Dodson based the indications for additional imaging of the mandibular third molar region when one or more of the high-risk radiographic findings described by Rood and colleagues were evident. According to Rood and colleagues,

Box 3. Use of panographs in the diagnosis and treatment planning of third molars

Identify the presence of third molars
Locate unusual position
Facilitate establishing their angulation
Show the vertical relationship to the
  second molar,
Identify caries and dentoalveolar bone
  loss
Detect the location of the inferior canal
Detect bone pathology
Establish the height of the mandible
Show the relationship of upper third
  molars and the maxillary sinus
Identify the structural stability of the
  second molar
Locate the relationship of root apices
  with dense bone
Detect dilacerated roots

concerns for increased risk of IAN damage should be heightened when there following conditions are present: (1) superimposition of the IAN canal and the third molar with narrowing of the IAN canal (Fig. 4), (2) darkening of the third molar root (Fig. 5), and (3) diversion of the IAN canal or loss of the white cortical outlines of the IAN (Fig. 6). When one or more of these findings is present, the risk of IAN damage ranges from 1.4% to 12%, with the baseline risk of IAN injury averaging approximately 1%. Dodson suggested periapical films or CT as reasonable imaging alternatives and cited evidence that absent any of the radiographic signs noted previously, the risk of IAN injury is low (<1%). CT imaging of third molar plays a role when the risk of IAN injury is high and there is sufficient evidence that third molar surgery is indicated.

Locating the lingual nerve clinically and by imaging is more problematic. Lingual nerve injury, although less common after third molar surgery than IAN injury using a buccal approach, is often more debilitating to the unfortunate patient [36]. Loss of taste, slurred speech, and tongue trauma are much less tolerated and adapted to by patients than IAN disturbances [37]. The anatomic positioning of the lingual nerve in the mouth floor is variable. Pogrel and colleagues [38] evaluated the relationship of third molar to the lingual nerve in 20 cadaveric (40) sides. The position of the nerve on one side did not have a statistical relationship to the position of the nerve on the opposite side. Variability in position of the lingual nerve was present in the sagittal and coronal planes. In two specimens, the nerve was located superior to the lingual plate and in another specimen the superior surface of the nerve was level with the crest of the lingual plate. Imaging of the lingual nerve is rarely necessary in

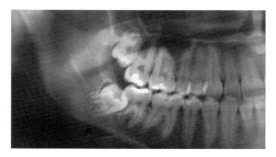

Fig. 4. Right mandibular third molar with roots that are intimately related to a narrowed inferior alveolar canal.

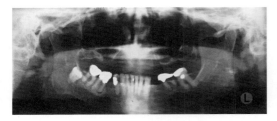

Fig. 5. Right asymptomatic mandibular third molar with roots that cross the inferior alveolar canal. Note that the apical third of the third molar root appears dark.

preparation for third molar surgery. Absent the bony canal that supports the IAN and marks it course on imaging studies, locating the lingual nerve is best done using MRI. Avoiding a lingual approach to third molar removal reduces the risk of lingual nerve injury [39].

Assessment of risk

Risk assessment associated with third molar surgery traditionally focuses on potential short- and long-term untoward sequela to the patient after surgery. Postoperative complications and their frequency, such as bleeding, persistent pain, dry socket, infection, altered sensation, trismus, dehydration, fractured jaw, and oral-antral communication, are explained to patients before the operative consent is signed. Should the risks to the surgeon and the surgical team also be considered? Should the findings of multiple HRQOL studies that indirectly offer the risks to employers, schools, and families of patients be considered when planning third molar surgery? How important to society is lost time from work or school, lost consortium, and protracted postoperative courses interfering with gainful activity? It is

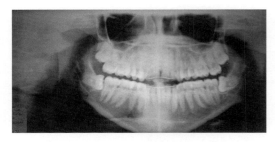

Fig. 6. Right mandibular third molar with roots that are associated with a curving inferior alveolar canal with loss of cortical outline.

prudent and necessary to consider risk assessment for third molar treatment for three interrelated constituencies: the patient, the operating team, and society.

Contemporary society's "need to know" is no longer limited to a description of potential or more likely complications of a surgical procedure. Patients demand more choices in their health care decisions and require a higher level of understanding before consenting to treatment. Presurgical considerations are important to patients and their family, employers, and other patient-ssociated affiliations (eg, school, sports teams, social interactions). Patients want to know about the surgical procedure and what they can expect during recovery. When will the patient be able to return to gainful activities? When can the patient return to work or school? Little information was previously available that documented patient perceptions of recovery after third molar surgery. The HRQOL studies previously cited provide a useful overview of patient perceptions after surgery [25,26].

Two hundred forty-nine patients (aged 13–37 years) at two clinical centers were enrolled in a prospective study before the surgical removal of third molars. Each patient was given a 21-item HRQOL instrument to be completed each postoperative day (POD) for 14 days. The instrument was designed to assess patients' perception of recovery: pain, oral function, general activity measures, and other symptoms. Pain dimensions were recorded with a seven-point Likert-type scale; all other conditions were measured on five-point Likert-type scales. The impact of each predictor variable (eg, age, gender, and length of surgery on recovery) was assessed statistically, controlling for clinical center. The results of the study can be useful to surgeons and patients when perioperative considerations of third molar surgery are discussed. Postoperatively most patients can expect to have their worst pain on POD 1, with the expectation by POD 7 that they have a 15% chance of experiencing their worst pain. Patients can be alerted that they will experience a high frequency of oral dysfunction—chewing, 85%; mouth opening, 78.5%; and speaking, 37.5%—on POD 1. Oral function should improve substantially by POD 6. Third molar surgery interferes with the lifestyle of most patients on POD 1 (social activity, 61.5%; recreation, 70.5%; daily routine, 60%), with most patients assuming a more normal life by POD 5. Swelling maximizes on POD 1 and 2. Patients should be informed that food collection in the surgical sites may pose a problem on POD 9.

In a second study, patients who were having four third molars removed were enrolled in an institutional review board–approved prospective clinical trial to assess clinical and HRQOL outcomes after surgery. A standard protocol (duplicating the 1999 study) maintained across multiple clinical centers included procedures common to surgery in the United States, such as intravenous anesthesia, access to the third molars from the buccal aspect, and bone removal for lower third molars with rotary instruments. During the 5 years of the study, from 1997 to 2001, 740 enrolled patients had their third molars removed. Every region in the country was represented except the southwest. Clinical and HRQOL data for recovery were available from 630 of the enrolled patients. The median age of the 630 patients who provided recovery data was 21 years. Bone removal at surgery was required for lower third molars in 33% of the patients; an additional 31% had bone removed in all third molars. Surgeons estimated the degree of difficulty of the surgery at each third molar site. The median estimate for the surgeons' overall degree of difficulty at surgery was 12 out of a possible 28 points on the Likert-type scale (IQ-interquartile range, 9–16). Surgeons indicated that mandibular third molars were more difficult to remove (8/14) than were maxillary third molars (5/14).

Twenty-two percent of the 630 patients who reported recovery data received treatment during at least one postsurgical visit. Eleven percent of all patients had a dressing placed in a third molar extraction site at the first postsurgical visit; 11% of all patients received treatment during multiple visits. Patients reported that the worst postsurgical pain they experienced occurred on POD 1. Fifty-four percent described the worst pain they experienced during the first 24 hours as severe, but only 20% reported their average pain over that period as severe. On POD 1, almost all patients (96%) were taking analgesic medications for pain. By POD 7, 55% were still taking pain medications; 13% were still taking medication for pain on POD 14.

Surgery affected the lifestyle and oral function of most patients on the first POD. Half the patients reported "quite a bit" or "lots" of lifestyle changes on POD 1. The patterns of decline in the percentage experiencing problems with mouth opening, return to regular diet, and chewing were similar, with chewing lagging behind slightly during the first postoperative week.

Approximately one fourth of patients reported problems with talking on POD 1.

Thirty-three percent of patients reported "quite a bit" or "lots" of trouble with swelling and bleeding on POD 1; less than 20% complained of nausea. Less than 10% of respondents had difficulty with nausea on POD 2. Swelling peaked on POD 2, bothering 46% of patients "quite a bit" or "lots." Other complaints, such as bad taste/breath, bothered 35% of respondents on POD 1 and were still a problem for 11% by the end of the first week. Recovery—the median number of days to "little or none/no trouble" for all of the HRQOL measures except pain and return to regular diet—was reached within 5 days after surgery: lifestyle, 4 days; absence of other symptoms, 3 days; and return to regular diet, 7 days.

In a study of risk factors associated with prolonged recovery and delayed healing after third molars surgery, 547 subjects with HRQOL and clinical outcome data were analyzed [40]. Delayed clinical healing was indicated by a patient having at least one postsurgical visit with treatment. Risk assessment models for prolonged HRQOL recovery and delayed healing were developed using stepwise logistic regression analysis. Age older than 18 years, female gender, and occlusal plane position were statistically associated with prolonged recovery for early symptoms, oral function, and pain. Recovery for lifestyle was prolonged only if both lower third molars were below the occlusal plane before surgery. Age older than 18 years, female gender, prior symptoms related to the third molars, and the surgeon's perception of difficulty were statistically significant predictors of delayed clinical recovery.

Patient risk factors

Factors that contribute to risk assessment for the patient are contained in Box 4. Surgeons may find it useful to initially provide patients with an overview of the remote and more common untoward intraoperative and postoperative events related to third molar surgery and then review the heightened risks for individual patients. Patients frequently inquire about postoperative pain, when they can return to gainful activity, and other HRQOL issues previously discussed. For the average, lean, healthy teenager with four soft tissue impactions who has a body type, psychosocial makeup, and surgeon-friendly head and neck anatomy, there is a high likelihood

Box 4. Factors that contribute to risk assessment for patients

Age
Location of IAN
Body mass index
Drug history
Systemic conditions
Surgical access space
Tongue size
Anesthesia history
Maxillary sinus location
Root contour
Third molar position
Interincisal opening
Health of semond Molar
Bone mass and density

that the surgery will proceed rapidly with minimal postoperative sequela. By contrast, the obese older patient with four full bony impacted third molars, dense bone, and dilacerated roots intimately associated with the inferior alveolar canal sleep apnea is more likely to experience more intraoperative trauma and a protracted postoperative course. Based on the surgical and patient factors of the individual case, the surgeon can emphasize the increased risks (eg, lost lip sensation when the inferior alveolar canal loses its radiographic margins at the apex of third molar). Advising high-risk patients that they should expect a longer more painful and life-interfering postoperative course is prudent and informative.

Surgical team risk factors

Communicable diseases should not be the only risks to the surgical team that are considered when evaluating patients for third molar surgery. Repetitive physical activity (eg, third molar removal) can be deleterious to surgeons and their staff when physical and mental strains on the operating team accumulate over time. Patient factors (eg, obesity, poor anesthetic responders) that portend visibility and surgical access difficulties for the operating team should be considered during the preoperative visit.

Practice management considerations

Overweight and obese patients present oral and maxillofacial surgeons with anesthetic, surgical, practice ergonomics, and potential postoperative problems that distinguish heavy patients from other patient cohorts. The operative team must be alert to the increased potential for airway obstruction, poor surgical visibility and accessibility, and the influence of intercurrent diseases on intraoperative and postoperative outcomes. Large patients are not compatible with standard size office equipment (surgical chairs, monitoring cuffs, wheel chairs) that are designed for smaller patients. Patient flow in the ambulatory setting may be disrupted when slow-moving, physically impaired patients with poor intravenous access sites inordinately intrude on efficient caregiving. Transferring patients after anesthesia may invite injury to the patient and members of the operating team. In aggregate, the routine logistics of seating, preparing, treating, and discharging patients may substantially increase the time and resources necessary to meet the obese patient's needs. Loss of practice efficiency translates into economic disadvantages for the surgeon, which unfortunately adds another important issue to the business side of oral and maxillofacial health care. Establishing key historical and physical examination findings helps the operative team decide on the appropriateness of outpatient care in the private office setting.

Intraoperative considerations

Inherent to the safe and effective practice of surgery is the surgeon's ability to visualize and have ready access to the surgical site. Operations are more likely to proceed smoothly when the surgical team is comfortably positioned around the patient. Ten morbidly obese individuals were retrospectively reviewed to determine the technical problems and incidence of surgical complications associated with knee joint arthroscopy [41]. When compared with a cohort of patients of normal weight who were matched for age, sex, and surgical procedure, the morbidly obese patients had longer operative times ($P < 0.02$). The authors reported that larger patients could not be accommodated by standard equipment, which created technical problems. To ensure a thorough examination, a greater number of arthroscopy portals were necessary. Poor posture and excessive twisting and reaching added to poor visibility, which translated into increased risk of surgical misadventures, increased operating time, and physical and mental stress on the oral and maxillofacial surgical team. Shorter team members are particularly disadvantaged. Taller, obese patients with wide shoulders and long torsos present the greatest surgical access challenge in the office environment.

Societal risks

Clinical and laboratory investigations into the etiology and consequences of periodontitis continue to enhance our understanding of the pathogenesis of this disease and the associated consequences. Recent studies have suggested a relationship between the progression of cardiovascular disease, diabetes mellitus, and pregnancy outcomes. Retaining asymptomatic third molars may increase the risk of periodontitis in susceptible patients with the associated local and less-defined systemic consequences.

Recovery for most HRQOL measures after third molar surgery in young adult patients occurred within 5 days. Recovery from pain to the criterion of "little or none" was delayed relative to other HRQOL measures, howver. A relationship existed between the degree of difficulty of the surgery and postsurgical recovery. Overall, 22% of patients may be at risk for delayed clinical healing after surgery. The effects of protracted postoperative recovery after third molar surgery have an impact on a patient's employer, family life, and other gainful social and commercial interactions.

Summary

Retained third molars may have associated periodontal pathology, although patients may have no symptoms. The deleterious consequences of periodontal pathology may not be limited to the third molar region or a negative impact on oral health. Asymptomatic patients also may have carious third molars. Caries seems to be limited to patients who have previous caries experience, caries, or restorations in first or second molars.

Third molars should be considered for removal when there is clinical, radiographic or laboratory evidence of acute or chronic periodontitis, caries, pericoronitis, deleterious affects on second molars, or pathology. Third molars that are in the field of anticipated orthognathic surgery or are interfering with prosthodontic or orthodontic care also should be removed. Extremes of age, increased risk of jaw fracture, poor surgical access, systemic illness, and increased risk of intraoperative or postoperative

complications may be contraindications to wisdom teeth removal.

Radiographic findings of extreme locations of impacted teeth, dense bone, dilacerated roots, large, radiolucent lesions associated with impactions, and lower third molar apices lodged in cortical inferior border bone are predictive of more complex surgery. Panographic observations of superimposition of the IAN canal and the third molar with narrowing of the IAN canal, darkening of the third molar root, diversion of the IAN canal, and loss of the white cortical outline of the IAN canal are predictive of an increased risk of IAN injury. Additional imaging should be considered when plain radiographs suggest high risk for IAN injury.

Assessment of risks related to third molar observation or treatment should be explained to patients. Candidates for surgery should be made aware of their personal likelihood of experiencing risks that are common to third molar extractions. Should the decision be made not to remove third molars, patients must be apprised of the risks of failure to treat. In addition to the direct consequences of third molar surgery on health, an overview of HRQOL postoperative effects should be advanced to patients. Preoperatively the surgical team should assess the appropriateness of the planned third molar surgery in a private office setting. Patient factors that portend increased intraoperative risks, poor surgical access, and compromised chair-side positioning of the surgical team or difficult perioperative office logistics are indications for a non-office operation site.

Certain demographic and oral health conditions available to the surgeon before surgery and intraoperative circumstances are predictive of delayed recovery for HRQOL outcomes (eg, early symptoms, lifestyle, late symptoms, oral function, pain) and delayed clinical outcomes (at least one postsurgical visit with treatment) after third molar surgery. If a patient is older than 18 years, the odds are increased for prolonged recovery for early symptoms, late symptoms, and pain. Female patients with surgery times longer than 20 minutes are likely to experience more postsurgical pain. If a patient presents with both lower third molars below the occlusal plane, h he or she is more likely to experience prolonged recovery for most HRQOL domains. If bone is removed from both lower third molars at surgery, the odds are increased for a prolonged recovery for lifestyle and oral function. Female gender, surgery that exceeds 40 minutes, symptoms before surgery, and surgeon assessment of procedure as difficult all increase the odds of a delayed clinical recovery.

References

[1] Song F, O'Meara S, Wilson P, et al. The effectiveness and cost-effectiveness of prophylactic removal of wisdom teeth. Health Technol Assess 2000;4(15): 1–55.

[2] Hicks EP. Third molar management: a case against routine removal in adolescent and young adult orthodontic patients. J Oral Maxillofac Surg 1999; 57(7):831–6.

[3] Woodhouse B. What is the future of third molar removal? Removal of impacted third molars: is the morbidity worth the risk? Ann R Australas Coll Dent Surg 1996;13:162–3.

[4] Harradine M, Pearson M, Toth B. The effects of extractions of third molars on late lower incisor crowding. Br J Orthod 1998;25(2):117–22.

[5] Hugoson A, Kugelberg CF. The prevalence of third molars in a Swedish population, an epidemiological study. Comm Dental Health 1988;5:121–38.

[6] Blakey GH, Marciani RD, Haug RH, et al. Periodontal pathology associated with asymptomatic third molars. J Oral Maxillofac Surg 2002;60: 1227–33.

[7] White R, Madianos P, Offenbacher S, et al. Microbial complexes detected in the second/third molar region in patients with asymptomatic third molars. J Oral Maxillofac Surg 2002;60:1234–45.

[8] Offenbacher S, Lieff S, Boggess KA, et al. Maternal periodontitis and prematurity. Part I: Obstetric outcome of prematurity and growth restriction. Ann Periodontol 2001;6:164–74.

[9] Slade G, Ghezzi EM, Heiss G, et al. Relationship between periodontal disease and C-reactive protein among adults in the Atherosclerosis Risk in Communities study. Arch Intern Med 2003;163:1172–9.

[10] Elter JR, Champagne CM, Offenbacher S, et al. Relationship of periodontal disease and tooth loss to prevalence of coronary disease. J Periodontol 2004; 75:782–90.

[11] Kshirsagar A, Moss KL, Elter JR, et al. Periodontal disease is associated with renal insufficiency in the Atherosclerosis Risk in Communities (ARIC) study. Am J Kidney Dis 2005;45:650–7.

[12] Blakey G, Jacks M, Offenbacher S, et al. Progression of periodontal disease in the second/third molar region in subjects with asymptomatic third molars. J Oral Maxillofac Surg 2006;64:189–93.

[13] White R, Madianos P, Offenbacher S, et al. Microbial complexes detected in the second/third molar region in subjects with asymptomatic third molars. J Oral Maxillofac Surg 2002;60:1234–40.

[14] Elter J, Cuomo C, Offenbacher S, et al. Third molars associated with periodontal pathology in the Third National Health and Nutrition Examination Survey. J Oral Maxillofac Surg 2004;62:440–5.

[15] Shugars D, Jacks M, White R, et al. Occlusal caries in patients with asymptomatic third molars. J Oral Maxillofac Surg 2004;62:973–9.

[16] Shugars D, Elter J, Jacks T, et al. Incidence of occlusal dental caries in asymptomatic third molars. J Oral Maxillofac Surg 2005;63:341–6.

[17] Zhu S, Choi B, Kim H, et al. Relationship between the presence of unerupted mandibular third molars and fractures of the mandibular condyle. Int J Oral Maxillofac Surg 2005;34:382–5.

[18] Hanson B, Cummings P, Rivara F, et al. The association of third molars with mandibular angle fractures: a meta-analysis. J Can Dent Assoc 2004;70: 39–43.

[19] Iida S, Hassfeld S, Reuther T, et al. Relationship between the risk of mandibular angle fractures and the status of incompletely erupted mandibular third molars. J Craniomaxillofac Surg 2005;33:158–63.

[20] Adeyemo W. Impacted lower third molars: another evidence against prophylactic removal. Int J Oral Maxillofac Surg 2005;34:816–7.

[21] Baykul T, Saglam A, Aydin U, et al. Incidence of cystic changes in radiologically normal impacted lower third molar follicles. Oral Surg Oral Med Oral Pathol Oral Radiol Endod 2005;99:542–5.

[22] National Institutes of Health. Removal of third molars: consensus statement. Bethesda (MD): National Institutes of Health; 1979. p. 65–8.

[23] Gibbons R. Germs, Dr. Billings and the theory of focal infection. Clin Infect Dis 1998;27:627–33.

[24] Kaminishi R, Lam P, Kaminishi K, et al. A 10-year comparative study of incidence of third molar removal in the aging population. J Oral Maxillofac Surg 2006;64(2):173–4.

[25] Conrad S, Blakey G, Shugars D, et al. Patients' perception of recovery after third molar surgery. J Oral Maxillofac Surg 1999;57:1288–94.

[26] White R, Shugars D, Shafer D, et al. Recovery after third molar surgery: clinical and health related quality of life outcomes. J Oral Maxillofac Surg 2003;61: 535–44.

[27] Peterson LJ. Principles of management of impacted teeth. In: Peterson LJ, Indresano AT, Marciani RD, et al, editors. Principles of oral and maxillofacial surgery. Philadelphia: JB Lippincott; 1992. p. 103–24.

[28] Pell G, Gregory B. Impacted third molars: classification and modified techniques for removal. Dent Dig 1933;39:330.

[29] Winter G. Impacted mandibular third molar. St. Louis (MO): American Medical Book Co.; 1926.

[30] Marciani R, Raezer B, Marciani H. Obesity and the practice of oral and maxillofacial surgery. Oral Surg Oral Med Oral Pathol Oral Radiol Endod 2004;98:10–5.

[31] Ford E, Giles W, Dietz W. Prevalence of the metabolic syndrome among US adults. JAMA 2002; 287:356–9.

[32] Pedersen G. Surgical removal of teeth. In: Surgical removal of teeth. Philadelphia: Pedersen; 1988. p. 63.

[33] Diniz-Freitas M, Lago-Mendez L, Gude-Sampedro F, et al. Pedersen scale fails to predict how difficult it will be to extract lower third molars. Br J Oral Maxillofac Surg 2006; in press.

[34] Dodson T. Role of computerized tomography in management of impacted mandibular third molars. N Y State Dent J 2005;71(6):32–5.

[35] Rood J, Nooraldeen Shehab B. The radiologic prediction of inferior alveolar nerve injury during third molar surgery. Br J Oral Maxillofac Surg 1990; 28:20.

[36] Robert R, Bacchetti P, Pogrel M. Frequency of trigeminal nerve injuries following third molar removal. J Oral Maxillofac Surg 2005;63(6):732–5.

[37] Graff-Radford S, Evans R. Lingual nerve injury. Headache 2003;43(9):975–83.

[38] Pogrel M, Renaut A, Schmidt B, et al. The relationship of the lingual nerve to the mandibular third molar region: an anatomic study. J Oral Maxillofac Surg 1995;53(10):1178–81.

[39] Donoff R. Raising lingual flaps increases the risk of nerve damage. Evid Based Dent 1998;1:14.

[40] Phillips C, White R, Shugars D. Risk factors associated with prolonged recovery and delayed healing after third molar surgery. J Oral Maxillofac Surg 2003;61(12):1436–48.

[41] Berg E. Knee joint arthroscopy in the morbidly obese. Arthroscopy 1999;15(2):321–4.

ELSEVIER
SAUNDERS

Oral Maxillofacial Surg Clin N Am 19 (2007) 15–21

ORAL AND
MAXILLOFACIAL
SURGERY CLINICS
of North America

Extraction Versus Nonextraction Management
of Third Molars

Shahrokh C. Bagheri, DMD, MD[a,b,]*, Husain Ali Khan, DMD, MD[b]

[a]Division of Oral and Maxillofacial Surgery, Emory University, Atlanta, GA, USA
[b]Private Practice, Atlanta Oral and Facial Surgery, Atlanta, GA, USA

In the United States, most practicing oral and maxillofacial surgeons routinely perform prophylactic removal of impacted third molars. The indications for removal of asymptomatic impacted third molars have been challenged [1–3]. This controversy has initiated the search for evidenced-based data to justify or dispute this practice. Do the risks and costs accumulated from the extraction of third molars outweigh the lifelong benefits obtained from their removal?

Decisions regarding this question not only should consider the presence of ongoing symptoms or pathology but also anticipate future complications and morbidity associated with retention of the third molars and possible increased risks of extraction at an older age. For modern health care policy determination, longitudinal studies using the tools of evidence-based medicine are necessary to address the full scope of factors influencing this decision. Individual clinical experience, opinions, personal bias, and individual financial motivations should have minimal influence on this decision. With the aging population, recent trends in health policy administration focus on prevention rather than treatment. Professional bodies recommending guidelines for the removal of impacted third molars also should focus on lifetime risks and benefits.

Two major professional organizations have made contradictory recommendations toward the prophylactic removal of impacted third molars. The American Association of Oral and Maxillofacial Surgeons (AAOMS) Third Molar Clinical Trials led by Dr. Raymond White published several scientific articles that link third molars to future health problems in adults. In light of these findings, in 2005, the AAOMS suggested that removing the third molars during young adulthood may be the most prudent option [4]. In contrast, the National Health Service of Great Britain and its associated arm, entitled the National Institute of Clinical Excellence, published a series of guidelines recommending that "The practice of prophylactic removal of pathology-free impacted third molars should be discontinued in the NHS" [1]. These guidelines, made public in 2000, acknowledged the ongoing AAOMS Third Molar Clinical Trials; however, as of the date of this writing, their recommendations remain to be revised to account for the more recently published evidence.

In this article we present the currently available evidence against and in support of the prophylactic removal of impacted third molars.

Evidence against prophylactic removal of third molars

In 2005, Mattes and colleagues [5] published a study that examined available randomized or controlled clinical trials supporting the removal of impacted third molars in young adults. They searched several databases, including Medline and Pubmed, from 1966 to 2004. They identified only three clinical trials that satisfied their search criteria. In their review of the literature they found no evidence to support or refute prophylactic removal of asymptomatic third molars in young adults [5].

* Corresponding author. 200 Galleria Parkway, Suite 1810, Atlanta, GA 30339.
E-mail address: sbagher@hotmail.com (S.C. Bagheri).

1042-3699/07/$ - see front matter © 2007 Elsevier Inc. All rights reserved.
doi:10.1016/j.coms.2006.11.009

In 2004, Iida and colleagues [3] reported a significant association between removal of impacted lower mandibular molars and mandibular condyle fractures. Subsequently, in 2005, Zhu and colleagues [2] also studied the relationship between the presence of unerupted mandibular third molars and fractures of the condyle. In this retrospective study of 439 mandibular fractures, they provided evidence suggesting that the removal of unerupted mandibular third molars predisposes to fractures of the condyle [2]. These two studies provided strong evidence to support that retention of the mandibular third molars help prevent fractures of the condyle.

Most young adults experience some degree of anterior mandibular incisor crowding, usually coinciding with the emergence of the third molars [6]. In 1996, Richardson [7] conducted a review of the literature that concluded that pressure from the posterior arch is an important cause of late mandibular incisor crowding. Among the many possible variables contributing to incisor crowding (eg, physiologic mesial drift, occlusal forces on mesially inclined teeth, mesial vectors of muscle contraction, developing third molars, mandibular and complex facial growth patterns, soft tissue maturation, occlusal factors, and connective tissue changes), it becomes difficult to design a study that can isolate all variables and demonstrate a cause-and-effect relationship between mandibular third molars and incisor crowding [8]. Many studies have attempted to demonstrate this causal relationship. A review of the available literature shows that most recent studies have not been able determine a relationship between mandibular third molars and anterior incisor crowding [9–15]. There seems to be no conclusive evidence to suggest that mandibular third molars should be extracted for prevention of late incisor crowding. In a more recent review by Zachrisson [16], he concludes that the available scientific evidence supports that the presence of a developing mandibular third molar with insufficient space can be one cause of late mandibular crowding. He suggests that the current studies fail to isolate third molars from all the other etiologic factors and cannot support the conclusion. Subsequently, some clinicians may advocate the removal of third molars to prevent anterior incisor crowding.

Several authors have suggested the increased incidence of complications with extraction of third molars with advancing age, including mandibular fractures [17] or trigeminal nerve injuries [18–21]. Haug and colleagues [22] recently conducted

a well-designed prospective study that evaluated 3760 patients aged 25 years who were undergoing removal of third molars by practicing oral and maxillofacial surgeons in the United States. The findings of this study indicated that third molar surgery in patients aged 25 years or older is associated with minimal morbidity, a low incidence of postoperative complications, and minimal impact on the patients' quality of life [22]. This study suggests that early extraction of third molars in young adulthood may not be necessary to prevent complications from potential extractions at an older age; however, the study does not focus on the elderly population.

Extraction of mandibular third molars is associated with a documented risk of injury to the lingual and inferior alveolar nerve. A recent study by Roberts and colleagues [23] examined reports of the frequency of temporary and permanent inferior alveolar and lingual nerve damage from lower third molar extractions by 535 California oral and maxillofacial surgeons. They found an overall self-reported rate of injury of 1 per 250 for lingual nerve and 1 per 1000 for inferior alveolar nerve (temporary and permanent). They reported rates of 1 per 2500 and 1 per 10,000 for permanent inferior alveolar nerve and lingual nerve injuries, respectively. The exact frequency of these complications is hard to determine accurately, however. Current publications report a significant variation from 0.5% to 5% for the inferior alveolar nerve and 0.6% to 2% for the lingual nerve [24–29]. If asymptomatic impacted mandibular third molars are found to bear no future oral or systemic health risks, it would be unnecessary to put a patient at risk for lingual or inferior alveolar nerve injury.

Finally, the guidelines from the National Institute of Clinical Excellence published initially in 2000 recommended against the prophylactic removal of impacted third molars in the British National Health Service [1]. Interpretation of the National Institute of Clinical Excellence guidelines should take into account that most third molar extractions in the United Kingdom are performed in a hospital setting. This approach is in contrast to the office-based procedure using intravenous anesthesia techniques, which is safely and widely practiced in the United States [30]. In the development of National Institute of Clinical Excellence guidelines, the added cost of outpatient general anesthesia for the National Health Service and the increased amount of time, resources, and personnel used to perform the same procedure must be accounted. In essence, the economics of third molar extractions are entirely different between the United Kingdom and the United States. This distinction brings different bearings on general health care policy determination for third molar extractions. In the ideal world, cost would not carry a significant weight for health care decisions. In reality, health policy and guidelines should account for resource use and provide the most effective health care given the available resources.

Evidence in support of prophylactic removal of third molars

In addition to the AAOMS Third Molar Clinical Trials, we reviewed the current literature regarding the evidence supporting the prophylactic extraction of third molars in early adulthood. It is important to evaluate the evidence regarding short-term (perioperative) and long-term complications from extraction of third molars. More importantly, the benefits of early extraction in regards to future complications, such as periodontal disease, systemic inflammation (and associated complications), mandibular fractures, development of cyst and tumors, odontogenic infections, anterior incisor crowding, and complications associated with extractions with advancing age, should be acknowledged.

Extensive evidence in the literature supports the fact that removing impacted third molars reduces the incidence of mandibular angle fractures [31–36], which is hypothesized to be caused by the decreased cross-sectional area of bone at the angle with a retained third molar and a greater susceptibility to mandibular angle fractures. A recent study by Wagner and colleagues [17] examined the clinical characteristics of pathologic mandibular angle fractures after third molar surgery. In their study group of 17 patients, 14 fractures occurred postoperatively and 16 (94%) fractures occurred in patients over the age of 40. According to these studies, extraction of third molars in young adulthood would reduce the incidence of mandibular angle fractures and prevent the relatively increased likelihood of a pathologic fracture if the procedure were to be performed at an older age.

It is generally accepted that third molars with associated pericoronal or periapical pathology should be extracted. Asymptomatic and radiographically pathology-free retained third molars do possess the potential of cystic (or neoplastic)

transformation over the lifespan of a patient, however. A recent study by Baykul and colleagues [37] investigated cystic changes in radiographically normal follicles associated with impacted lower third molars. The authors concluded that cystic changes may be encountered in the histopathologic examination of asymptomatic third molars, especially in patients older than 20 years of age (50% of patients). Another study by Salgam and Tuzum [38] reported an incidence of complications, such as pain, cysts, resorption of adjacent teeth, infection, crowding, and changes in position of the adjacent teeth, in more than 28% of their study group. The authors recommended the extraction of fully impacted third molars before the onset of complications. They acknowledged the economic restraints in socioeconomically poor populations. Other previous studies have confirmed a high proportion of soft tissue pathologic conditions for asymptomatic third molars [39–41]. Glosser and Campbell [41] examined the incidence of histologic abnormalities in soft tissue surrounding impacted third molar teeth in the absence of radiographic signs of pathology. They identified dentigerous cysts in 37% of mandibular and 25% of maxillary impacted third molars. In a similar study (n = 100), Adelsperger and colleagues [39] reported a 34% incidence of squamous metaplasia, which suggested cystic change equivalent to that found in dentigerous cysts. Rakprasitikul [40] also studied the incidence of pathologic changes associated with unerupted third molars in 104 patients. He found normal dental follicles in 41% of patients, with an incidence of pathologic changes in 59% (dentigerous cyst, 51.0%; chronic nonspecific inflammation, 4.8%; odontogenic keratocysts, 1.9%).

The early extraction of third molars eliminates the need for future, more extensive surgical treatments at an older age should a pathologic condition develop. With a high incidence of pathologic changes in third molars with normal radiographic appearance, prevention of aggressive odontogenic cysts (eg, dentigerous or odontogenic keratocysts) becomes a significant benefit of early extraction of third molars. Similarly, odontogenic tumors that arise from impacted third molars bear similar implications. These tumors have a much smaller incidence, however. In the study by Rakprasitikul [40], the incidence of ameloblastoma in association with the impacted third molar was less than 1%. the treatment of such tumors is frequently associated with much greater morbidity and disability.

The effects of extraction versus retention of asymptomatic impacted third molars on the periodontal health of the adjacent second molar have shown some conflicting results. Earlier studies have suggested that extraction of impacted third molars can cause deepening of the periodontal defects distal to the second molar [42–44]. In contrast, several authors have shown improvement in periodontal attachment levels after third molar extraction [45–50]. In 2005, Richardson and Dodson [51] conducted a well-designed report using evidence-based principles to evaluate the risk of periodontal defects after third molar surgery. They conducted a computerized search to identify relevant articles (using Medline) for prospective cohort or randomized clinical trials with adequate follow-up (>6 months). In this comprehensive review of the literature, they concluded that most commonly the second molar attachment levels or periodontal depths either remain unchanged or improved after third molar extraction. They did find, however, that given a healthy preoperative periodontal status, 48% of patients have worsening of their periodontal status after removal of the third molars [51]. There is strong evidence that pre-existing periodontal disease around the distal of the second molar generally improves with extraction of the third molars.

The findings of the AAOMS Third Molars Clinical Trials have demonstrated new evidence linking periodontal disease with systemic effects in young adults. Studies have linked oral bacteria associated with periodontal disease with serious health problems, such as coronary artery disease, stroke, renal vascular disease, diabetes, and obstetric complications [52–55]. Offenbacher and colleagues [56] recently published a study that examined periodontal disease and the risk of preterm delivery. They studied 1020 pregnant women who received antepartum and postpartum periodontal examinations. The conclusions clearly demonstrate that maternal periodontal disease increases the relative risk of preterm or spontaneous preterm births. Mothers with third molar periodontal pathology had elevated serum markers of systemic inflammation (C-reactive protein, isoprostanes). Periodontal disease was also a predictor of more severe adverse pregnancy outcomes.

A key finding in the Third Molar Clinical Trials is evidence suggesting that untreated periodontal disease provides a portal of entry for pathogenic bacteria into the bloodstream [57]. The data indicate that patients with periodontal attachment loss have increased levels of biochemical markers of inflammation compared with controls [57]. In subsequent studies, the association of third molars with periodontal pocketing [58] and the progression and presence of periodontitis in the third molar region in asymptomatic patients was elucidated [59,60]. In another study, White and colleagues [61] examined microbial colonization in the second/third molar region in patients with asymptomatic third molars. The study supported that microbial changes associated with the initiation of periodontitis may present first in the third molar region in young adults. The Third Molar Clinical Trials suggest that most third molars, even those that are asymptomatic and display no current signs of disease, should be considered for removal in young adulthood.

What is the lifetime incidence of deep facial space or odontogenic infections (pericoronitis, osteomyelitis) in patients with retained asymptomatic third molars? The answer to this question requires longitudinal studies of patients with asymptomatic impacted third molars that are monitored prospectively for the development of infections. Until such studies are available, this question cannot be resolved conclusively. The presentation of an infected third molar with its associated morbidity in the elderly population, who commonly present with other medical conditions along with multiple medications (eg, bisphosphonates, anticoagulants, chemotherapeutic agents), can be challenging, however. Osaki and colleagues [62] studied infections in elderly patients associated with impacted third molars. They looked at 41 patients older than 60 years of age (26 cases of pericoronitis, 8 infected dentigerous cysts, 4 mandibular abscesses, 2 chronic osteomyelitis, 1 odontogenic fistula) and outlined some of the challenges pertaining to the treatment of these conditions in the elderly population. Kunkel and colleagues [63] conducted a 1-year prospective study of third molar extractions requiring in-patient hospitalization. In their sample of patients, they found that infectious complications were the most frequent and more severe and required more extensive hospitalizations and treatment. They noticed that the complications from prophylactic removal at a young age were significantly less than extraction of symptomatic teeth at an older age [63]. Their data support extraction of impacted third molars with the goal of preventing future serious infections. Yoshii and colleagues [64] examined 993 patients who underwent third molar extractions. Although the incidence of deep facial space infections after the removal of mandibular third molars was low (0.8%), they recommended the extraction of third molars at an earlier age because of the higher incidence of infections in patients over the age of 30. The greater degree of complications associated with extraction of third molars in elderly persons may be avoided by early extraction of third molars with minimal associated morbidity.

Extraction of third molars is associated with a risk of injury to the inferior alveolar or lingual nerve. Proponents of nonextraction may argue that this would be an unnecessary risk in a pathology-free state. Future pathologic conditions cannot be predicted in young adulthood, however. Pathologic conditions related to the third molars (eg, periodontal disease, infection, tumors, or cysts) can develop at a later age and require extraction. The incidence of nerve injuries is statistically associated with the age of the patient [65,66], which is partially related to the chronology of third molar development. The roots of the third molars are usually not fully formed until age 21. Subsequently, extraction of third molars in the teenage years is associated with a lower incidence of inferior alveolar nerve injury. The greater regenerative capacity of younger adults is associated with a greater chance of recovery with nerve injuries [67]. Extraction of the third molars at an earlier age could decrease the incidence of inferior alveolar and lingual nerve injuries.

A possible link between extraction of third molars and internal derangement of the temporomandibular joint has been suggested [68]; however, it has not been confirmed by other authors. In 2005, Threlfall and colleagues [69] conducted a case controlled study that examined a series of 220 patients with temporomandibular joint anterior disc displacement with reduction. They found that patients with disc displacement are not significantly more likely to have had extraction of third molars than controls. They concluded that extraction of third molars is unlikely to be a cause of temporomandibular joint disc displacement with reduction. No conclusive evidence supports extraction of third molars as a cause of chronic temporomandibular joint disorders.

Summary

Although in some regions of the world socioeconomic and available resources play a greater role in determining guidelines for third molar extractions, the current scientific evidence remains unchanged. The cumulative financial costs of treating the health complications of retained third molars in the older population should be accounted. Although it is clear that extraction of third molars pose some risks to the patients, determination of extraction versus nonextraction of asymptomatic third molars should compare the cost and risks of surgical extraction to the lifetime health and cost benefits from prevention and elimination of any pathologic processes associated with retention of the third molars.

The effectiveness, safety, and relatively minimal cost incurred by extraction of third molars using outpatient office-based anesthesia along with currently available scientific evidence linking asymptomatic third molars to multiple health hazards overwhelmingly supports the extraction of asymptomatic third molars in young adulthood.

References

[1] National Institute for Clinical Excellence. Guidance on the extraction of wisdom teeth. Available at: http://www.nice.org.uk/pdf/wisdomteethguidance.pdf. Accessed March 9, 2006.

[2] Zhu SJ, Chi BH, Kim HJ, et al. Relationship between the presence of unerupted mandibular third molars and fractures of the mandibular condyle. Int J Oral Maxillofac Surg 2005;34:382–5.

[3] Iida S, Nomura K, Okura M, et al. Influence of the incompletely erupted lower third molar on mandibular angle and condylar fractures. J Trauma 2004;57:613–7.

[4] American Association of Oral and Maxillofacial Surgeons. News release: research study links wisdom teeth to health problems in young adults. Rosemont (IL): American Association of Oral and Maxillofacial Surgeons; 2005.

[5] Mattes TG, Nienhuijs ME, van der Sanden WJ, et al. Interventions for treating asymptomatic impacted wisdom teeth in adolescents and adults. Cochrane Database Syst Rev 2005;18(2):CD003879.

[6] Sampson WJ. Current controversies in late incisor crowding. Ann Acad Med Singapore 1995;24(1):129–37.

[7] Richardson ME. The etiology of late lower arch crowding alternative to mesially directed forces. Am J Orthod Dentofacial Orthop 1994;105:592–7.

[8] Richardson ME. Late lower arch crowding in relation to skeletal and dental morphology and growth changes. Br J Orthod 1996;23:249–54.

[9] Buschang PH, Shulman JD. Incisor crowding in untreated persons 15–50 years of age: United States, 1988–1994. Angle Orthod 2003;73(5):502–8.

[10] Little RM. Stability and relapse of mandibular anterior alignment: University of Washington studies. Semin Orthod 1999;5(3):191–204.

[11] Harradine NW, Pearson MH, Toth B. The effect of extraction of third molars on late lower incisor crowding: a randomized controlled trial. Br J Orthod 1998;25(2):117–22.

[12] Vander der shoot EAM, Kulter RB, van Ginkel M, et al. Clinical relevance of third permanent molars in relation to crowding after orthodontic treatment. J Dent 1990;25:167–9.

[13] Pirttiniemi PM, Oikarienen KS, Raustia AM. The effect of removal of all third molars on the dental arches in the third decade of life. Cranio 1994; 12(1):23–7.

[14] Ades AG, Joondeph DR, Little RM, et al. A long term study of the relationship of third molars changes in the mandibular dental arch. Am J Orthod Dentofacial Orthop 1990;97:323–35.

[15] Kaplan RG. Mandibular third molars and post-retention crowding. Am J Orthod 1976;70:147–53.

[16] Zachrisson BU. Mandibular third molars and late lower arch crowding: the evidence base. World J Orthod 2005;6(2):180–6.

[17] Wagner KW, Otten JE, Schoen R, et al. Pathological mandibular fractures following third molar removal. Int J Oral Maxillofac Surg 2005;34(7):722–6.

[18] Kipp DP, Goldstein BH, Weiss WW. Dysesthesia after mandibular third molar surgery: a retrospective study and an analysis of 1377 surgical procedures. J Am Dent Assoc 1980;100:1985.

[19] Bruce RA, Friederickson GC, Small GS. Age of patients and morbidity associated with mandibular third molar surgery. J Am Dent Assoc 1980;101:240.

[20] Fielding AF, Douglass AF, Whitely RD. Reasons for early removal of impacted third molars. Clin Prev Dent 1981;3:19.

[21] Osborne TP, Frederickson G, Small IA, et al. A prospective study of complications related to mandibular third molar surgery. J Oral Maxillofac Surg 1985; 43:767.

[22] Haug RH, Perrott DH, Gonzalez ML, et al. The American Association of Oral and Maxillofacial Surgeons age-related third molar study. J Oral Maxillofac Surg 2005;63:1106–14.

[23] Roberts RC, Bacchetti P, Pogrel MA. Frequency of trigeminal nerve injuries following third molar removal. J Oral Maxillofac Surg 2005;63:732–5.

[24] Alling CC III. Dysesthesia of the lingual and inferior alveolar nerves following third molar surgery. J Oral Maxillofac Surg 1986;44:454.

[25] Goldberg MH, Nemarich AN, Marco WP. Complications after mandibular third molar surgery: a statistical analysis of 500 consecutive procedures in private practice. J Am Dent Assoc 1985;11:277.

[26] Kipp DP, Goldstein BH, Weiss WW Jr. Dysesthesia after mandibular third molar surgery: a retrospective study and analysis of 1,377 surgical procedures. J Am Dent Assoc 1980;100:185.

[27] Merrill RG. Prevention, treatment and prognosis for nerve injury related to the difficult impaction. Dent Clin North Am 1979;23:471.

[28] Osborn TP, Frederickson G Jr, Small IA, et al. A prospective study of complications related to mandibular third molar surgery. J Oral Maxillofac Surg 1985;43:767.

[29] Wolford DT, Miller RI. Prospective study of dysesthesia following odontectomy of impacted mandibular third molars. J Oral Maxillofac Surg 1987;43:15.

[30] Perrott DH, Yuen JP, Andresen RV, et al. Office-based ambulatory anesthesia: outcomes of clinical practice of oral and maxillofacial surgeons. J Oral Maxillofac Surg 2003;61(9):983–95.

[31] Schwimmer A, Stern R, Kritchman D. Impacted third molars: a contributory factor in mandibular fractures in contact sports. Am J Sports Med 1983; 11:262–6.

[32] Sadfar N, Meechan JG. Relationship between fractures of the mandible angle and the presence and state of eruption of the lower third molars. Oral Surg Oral Med Oral Pathol Oral Radiol Enodod 1995;79:680–4.

[33] Ugboko VI, Oginni FO, Owotade FJ. An investigation into the relationship between mandibular third molars and angle fractures in Nigerians. Br J Oral Maxillofac Surg 2000;38:427–9.

[34] Hanson BP, Cummings P, Rivara FP, et al. The association of third molars with mandibular angle fractures: a meta-analysis. J Can Dent Assoc 2004; 70:39–43.

[35] Iida S, Nomura K, Okura M, et al. Influence of the incompletely erupted third molar on mandibular angle fractures. J Trauma 2004;57:613–7.

[36] Iida S, Hassefeld S, Reuther T, et al. Relationship between the risk of mandibular angle fractures and the status of incompletely erupted mandibular third molars. J Craniomaxillofac Surg 2005;33:158–63.

[37] Baykul T, Saglam AA, Ulkem A, et al. Incidence of cystic changes in radiographically normal impacted lower third molar follicles. Oral Surg Oral Med Oral Pathol Oral Radiol Endod 2005;99:542–5.

[38] Salgam AA, Tuzum MS. Clinical and radiologic investigation of the incidence, complications, and suitable removal times for fully impacted teeth in the Turkish population. Quintessence Int 2003; 34(1):53–9.

[39] Adelsperger J, Campbell JH, Coates DB, et al. Early soft tissue pathosis associated with impacted third molars without pericoronal radiolucency. Oral Surg Oral Med Oral Pathol Oral Radiol Endod 2000;89(4):402–6.

[40] Rakprasitikul S. Pathologic changes in the pericoronal tissues of unerupted third molars. Quintessence Int 2001;32(8):633–8.

[41] Glosser JW, Campbell JH. Pathologic change in soft tissues associated with radiographically normal third molar impactions. Br J Oral Maxillofac Surg 1999;37(4):259–60.

[42] Ash MM Jr, Costich ER, Hayward JR. A study of periodontal hazards of third molars. J Periodontol 1962;33:209–19.

[43] Zeigler RS. Preventive dentistry: new concepts: preventing periodontal pockets. Va Dent J 1975;52: 11–3.

[44] Kugelberg Ahlstrom U, Ericson S, Hugoson A. Periodontal healing after impacted lower third molar surgery: a retrospective study. Int J Oral Surg 1985;44:29–40.

[45] Szmyd L, Hester WR. Crevicular depth of the second molar in impacted third molar surgery. J Oral Surg 1963;21:185–9.

[46] Grondahl HG, Lekholm U. Influence of mandibular third molars on related supporting tissues. Int J Oral Surg 1973;2:137–42.

[47] Groves BJ, Moore JR. Periodontal implications of flap design in lower third molar extractions. Dent Pract Dent Rec 1970;20:297–304.

[48] Stephens RJ, App GR, Foreman DW. Periodontal evaluation of two mucoperiosteal flaps used in removing impacted mandibular third molars. J Oral Maxillofac Surg 1983;41:719–24.

[49] Wolf RH, Malmquist JP, Wright WH. Third molar extractions: periodontal implications of two flap designs. Gen Dent 1978;26:52–6.

[50] Krausz AA, Machtei EE, Peled M. Effects of lower third molar extraction on attachment level and alveolar bone height of the adjacent second molar. Int J Oral Maxillofac Surg 2005;34:756–60.

[51] Richardson DT, Dodson TD. Risk of periodontal defects after third molar surgery: an exercise in evidence-based clinical decision-making. Oral Surg Oral Med Oral Pathol Oral Radiol Endod 2005; 100(2):133–7.

[52] Offenbacher S, Elter JR, Lin D, et al. Evidence for periodontitis as a tertiary vascular infection. J Int Acad Periodontol 2005;7(2):39–48.

[53] Beck JD, Eke P, Lin D, et al. Associations between IgG antibody to oral organisms and carotid intima-medial thickness in community-dwelling adults. Atherosclerosis 2005;183(2):342–8.

[54] Beck JD, Elter J, Heiss G, et al. Relationship of periodontal disease to carotid artery intima-media wall thickness: the atherosclerosis risk in communities (ARIC) study. Arterioscler Thromb Vasc Biol 2001;21(11):1816–22.

[55] Elter JR, Hinderliter AL, Offenbacher S, et al. The effects of periodontal therapy on vascular endothelial function: a pilot trial. Am Heart J 2006; 151(1):47.

[56] Offrenbacher S, Boggess KA, Murtha AP, et al. Progressive periodontal disease and risk of very preterm delivery. Obstet Gynecol 2006;107(1):29–36.

[57] White RP, Offenbacher S, Phillips C, et al. Inflammatory mediators and periodontitis in patients with asymptomatic third molars. J Oral Maxillofac Surg 2002;60(11):1241–5.

[58] Elter JR, Offenbacher S, White RP Jr. Association of third molars with periodontal pocketing: the dental ARIC study. J Oral Maxillofac Surg 2004;62(Suppl 1):73–4.

[59] Blakey GH, Marciani RD, Haug RH, et al. Periodontal pathology associated with asymptomatic third molars. J Oral Maxillofac Surg 2002;60(11): 1227–33.

[60] Blakey GH, Jacks MT, Offenbacher S, et al. Progression of periodontal disease in the second/third molar region in subjects with asymptomatic third molars. J Oral Maxillofac Surg 2006;64(2):189–93.

[61] White RP Jr, Madianos PN, Offenbacher S, et al. Microbial complexes detected in the second/third molar region in patients with asymptomatic third molars. J Oral Maxillofac Surg 2002;60(11):1234–40.

[62] Osaki T, Nomura Y, Hirota J, et al. Infections in elderly patients associated with impacted third molars. Oral Surg Oral Med Oral Pathol Oral Radiol Endod 1995;79(2):137–41.

[63] Kunkel M, Morbach T, Wagner W. Wisdom teeth: complications requiring in-patient treatment. A 1-year prospective study. Mund Kiefer Gesichtschir 2004;8(6):44–9.

[64] Yoshii T, Hamamoto Y, Muraoka S, et al. Incidence of deep facial space infection after surgical removal of mandibular third molars. J Infect Chemother 2001;7(1):55–7.

[65] Queral-Gody E, Valmaseda-Castellon E, Berini-Aytes L, et al. Incidence and evolution of inferior alveolar nerve lesions following lower third molar extractions. Oral Surg Oral Med Oral Pathol Oral Radiol Endod 2005;99(3):259–64.

[66] Valmaseda-Castellon E, Berini-Aytes L, Gay-Escoda C. Inferior alveolar nerve damage after lower third molar surgical extraction: a prospective study of 1117 surgical extractions. Oral Surg Oral Med Oral Pathol Oral Radiol Endod 2001;92(4): 377–83.

[67] Dellon AL. Wound healing in nerve. Clin Plast Surg 1990;17:545.

[68] Huang GL, LeRosche L, Critchlow CW, et al. Risk factors for diagnostic subgroups of painful temporomandibular disorders (TMD). J Dent Res 2002;81: 284–8.

[69] Threlfall AG, Kanaa MD, Davies SJ, et al. Possible link between extraction of wisdom teeth and temporomandibular disc displacement with reduction: matched case control study. Br J Oral Maxillofac Surg 2005;43(1):13–6.

ORAL AND
MAXILLOFACIAL
SURGERY CLINICS
of North America

Oral Maxillofacial Surg Clin N Am 19 (2007) 23–43

General Technique of Third Molar Removal

Sam E. Farish, DMD[a,b,*],
Gary F. Bouloux, MD, BDS, MDSc, FRACDS, FRACDS(OMS)[b]

[a]Division of Oral and Maxillofacial Surgery, Atlanta Veterans Affairs Medical Center, Atlanta, GA, USA
[b]Division of Oral and Maxillofacial Surgery, Emory University School of Medicine, 1365B Clifton Road NE,
Suite 2300-B, Atlanta, GA 30322, USA

The most commonly performed surgical procedure in most oral and maxillofacial surgery practices is the removal of impacted third molars. Extensive training, skill, and experience allow this procedure to be performed in an atraumatic fashion with local anesthesia, sedation, or general anesthesia. The decision to remove symptomatic third molars is not usually difficult, but the decision to remove asymptomatic third molars is sometimes less clear and requires clinical experience. A wide body of literature (discussed elsewhere in this issue) attempts to establish clinical practice guidelines for dealing with impacted teeth [1]. Data are beginning to accumulate from third molar studies, which hopefully will provide surgeons and their patients with evidence-based guidelines regarding elective third molar surgery [2–6]. The association of periodontal pathology and occlusal caries with asymptomatic third molars has been studied previously. Twenty-five percent of patients with asymptomatic third molars were found to have increased periodontal probing depths and attachment loss, increased periodontal pathogen colonization, and increased levels of inflammatory mediators [7–9]. Shugars and colleagues [10] examined a group of patients with at least one fully erupted third molar and found that 28% had caries in at least one third molar tooth. It is currently recommended that the indications for elective therapeutic third molar removal be based on good clinical science. Accordingly, patients and the community at large should be adequately informed [11].

Once the decision is made to remove impacted third molars, a classification system based on clinical and radiographic findings becomes a tool for predicting the difficulty of removal. Accessibility significantly influences the degree of difficulty of removal of a third molar. The ease with which the tooth can be removed is also influenced by the degree of surgical exposure, the ability to create a pathway for tooth delivery, and the ability to gain purchase (natural or surgically prepared) on the tooth. A classification system is a useful tool to categorize the degree of impaction and plan a surgical approach that facilitates removal and minimizes morbidity.

Classification systems of impacted teeth

Most classifications of third molar impactions are based on the analysis of periapical—or more commonly, panoramic—radiographs. The initial determination that should be made is the angulation of the third molar to the long axis of the second molar. The mesioangular impaction, which accounts for approximately 43% of all mandibular impacted third molars, is one in which the third molar is mesially tilted toward the second molar [12]. Such impactions are generally considered the least difficult to remove (Fig. 1A).

An exaggerated mesial inclination results in a horizontal impaction (Fig. 1B), which is considered more difficult to remove than a mesioangular impaction and accounts for approximately 3% of all mandibular impactions [12]. The vertical impaction, in which the long axis of the impacted tooth runs parallel to the long axis of the second molar, is seen in approximately 38% of all mandibular impactions (Fig. 1C) [12]. It is considered

---

* Corresponding author.
 E-mail address: sefaris@emory.edu (S.E. Farish).

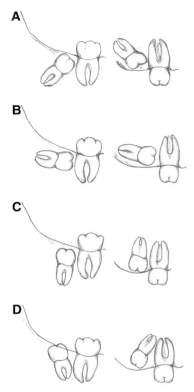

Fig. 1. Angulation classification system for impacted third molars. (*A*) Mesioangular lower and upper third molar impactions. (*B*) Horizontal lower and upper third molar impactions. (*C*) Vertical lower and upper third molar impactions. (*D*) Distoangular lower and upper third molar impactions.

more difficult than a mesioangular or horizontal impaction.

The distoangular impaction, in which the long axis of the impacted tooth is inclined distally (Fig. 1D), occurs uncommonly and accounts for approximately 6% of mandibular impactions but

is considered the most difficult impaction to remove [12]. The path of removal of this tooth is into the ramus and requires more extensive bone removal for its successful delivery. Erupted lower third molars also frequently are found with a distoangular inclination. Most mandibular third molars are also angled toward the lingual (in lingual version) because the lingual cortical plate progressively thins from anterior to posterior. Impacted mandibular third molars may be in buccal version, however, and rarely in a transversely oriented position. A transversely oriented unerupted tooth can be further evaluated with an occlusal film to disclose the position of the third molar in the coronal plane, but surgical exposure also rapidly allows determination of the tooth position [12].

The Pell and Gregory classification relates the position of the impacted mandibular third molar to the ramus of the mandible in an anterior-posterior direction [13]. When the mesiodistal diameter of the third molar crown is completely anterior to the anterior border of the ramus, it is considered a class 1 relationship (Fig. 2A). Such a tooth can be angled in a mesial, distal, or vertical direction. The likelihood for normal eruption is best for a class 1 tooth with a vertical angulation. In a Pell and Gregory class 2 relationship, approximately one half the mesiodistal diameter of the mandibular third molar is covered by the ramus of the mandible (Fig. 2B). The distal aspect of the crown of teeth in this position is covered by bone and soft tissue. Teeth so positioned are particularly susceptible to caries and pericoronitis.

A Pell and Gregory class 3 relationship involves an impacted mandibular third molar that is located completely within the ramus (Fig. 2C). The accessibility of a class 3 impaction is such that it should be considered the most difficult tooth to remove. A mandibular third molar in a class 1 relationship should not be difficult to

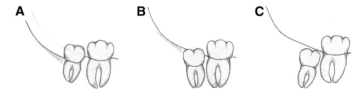

Fig. 2. Pell and Gregory classification based on relationship to the anterior border of the ramus. (*A*) Class 1 impaction, in which mandibular third molar has sufficient room anterior to the anterior border of the ramus to erupt. (*B*) Class 2, in which half of the impacted third molar is covered by the ramus. (*C*) Class 3, in which the impacted third molar is completely embedded in the ramus of the mandible.

remove, whereas a class 2 relationship would be more difficult than a class 1 relationship but less difficult than a class 3 relationship.

The vertical relationship of the occlusal surface of the impacted mandibular third molar to the occlusal plane of the second molar tooth is also described by the Pell and Gregory classification. The degree of difficulty in removing a mandibular third molar increases as the depth of the tooth below the occlusal plane of the second molar increases. As the depth of the impaction increases, the accessibility decreases and elevation, sectioning, and purchase point preparation become increasingly difficult. In a class A impaction, the occlusal surface of the third molar is at the same level as the occlusal plane of the second molar (Fig. 3A). In a class B impaction, the occlusal plane of the impacted tooth is between the occlusal plane and the cervical line of the second molar (Fig. 3B). A class C impaction results when the occlusal surface of the impacted third molar is below the cervical line of the second molar (Fig. 3C).

These classifications are used to determine the degree of the impaction and develop a plan for the removal of impacted third molars. A mesioangular impaction with a class 1 ramus and class A depth relationship would be the easiest type of impaction to remove (Fig. 4A). A distoangular impaction with a class 3 ramus relationship and a class C depth (Fig. 4B) would involve a difficult surgical procedure.

The classification system based on the dental procedure codes that are used by insurance carriers is also relevant for review [14]. These codes are based on clinical and radiographic interpretation of the tissue overlying the impacted maxillary or mandibular third molar. A D7220 is the removal of an impaction whose height of contour is above the alveolar bone and covered by soft tissue only—a soft tissue impaction (Fig. 5A). Such a removal is accomplished by incision and reflection of a soft tissue flap and elevation and is considered simple. A D7230 is the removal of an impaction whose superficial contour is covered by soft tissue and whose height of contour lies beneath the surrounding alveolar bone—a partial bony impaction (Fig. 5B). Such teeth are removed after a soft tissue flap, some bone removal, and possibly tooth sectioning. Surgeries coded D7230 are considered intermediate in difficulty in the spectrum of impacted third molar removal. When an impacted third molar is covered with soft tissue and bone, its removal is coded D7240—full bony impaction (Fig. 5C). Such teeth require soft-tissue flap elevation followed by removal of overlying bone and, frequently, sectioning of the tooth for removal. These impactions are considered the most difficult to remove. An additional code, D7241, can be used for complete bony impactions with unusual surgical complications (eg, root aberrations, proximity to anatomic structures, internal or external resorption) that make the removal of such teeth even more difficult than regular full bony impactions.

Root morphology also influences the degree of difficulty for removal of an impacted third molar. Limited root development leads to a "rolling" tooth, which can be difficult to remove. Such teeth are easier dealt with by sectioning in multiple planes before any mobility is obtained. A tooth with one-third to two-thirds root development is easier to remove than a tooth with full root development. Such teeth typically have a wide periodontal ligament, and ample space exists between the roots and the inferior alveolar nerve (IAN). Similarly, third molars with conical and fused roots are easier to remove than third molars with widely separated and distinct roots. Roots with severe curves, however, are more difficult to

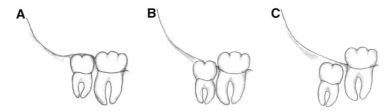

Fig. 3. Pell and Gregory classification based on relationship to the occlusal plane. (A) Class A impaction, in which the occlusal plane of the impacted tooth is the same as the second molar. (B) Class B, in which the occlusal plane of the impacted third molar is between the occlusal plane and the cervical line of the second molar. (C) Class C, in which the occlusal plane of the impacted third molar is below the cervical line of the second molar.

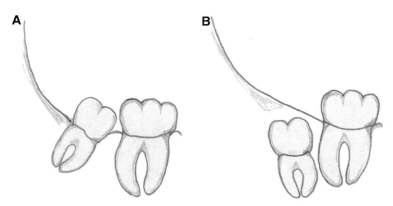

Fig. 4. Examples of combinations of angulation, anterior ramus, and occlusal plane classifications. (*A*) A mesioangular impaction with a class 1 ramus and class A depth relationship—an easy third molar impaction. (*B*) A distoangular impaction with a class 3 ramus and a class C depth—a difficult impaction.

remove than less curved or essentially straight roots. Roots that curve in the same direction as the pathway of removal break less often than roots that curve in a direction opposite to the pathway of removal. Roots with a mesiodistal diameter that is greater than the tooth diameter at the cervical line must be sectioned longitudinally (Fig. 6). Despite a Pell and Gregory classification of 1A, teeth that are erupted and functional often have a narrow periodontal ligament space, which makes elevator placement and mobility more difficult to achieve. Conversely, unerupted teeth with follicular sacs (younger patients) require less bone removal as a result of the wide periodontal ligament and a large coronal cavity secondary to the follicle [12].

When considering bone density, young patients are considered to have less dense bone than patients older than 35 years of age [12]. The more dense the bone, the less the degree of bony expansion during luxation and the more time required for its removal with a bur. The space between the distal surface of the second molar and the mesial surface of the impacted third also has an impact on the ease of removal of the third molar. The closer the third molar is to the second molar, the more difficult the surgery becomes. Large restorations, crowns, and root canal therapy in second molar teeth also pose additional risks of damage to the second molar if elevation forces or drilling vectors are misdirected. In cases in which crowns or large restorations exist in proximity to impacted or erupted third molars slated for removal, informed consent should be explicit regarding possible damage to an adjacent tooth.

The relationship of the mandibular third molar roots to the IAN must be considered when surgical removal is contemplated. Surgical planning and proper informed consent depend on detailed knowledge of the positional relationships in this area. The more intimate the relationship of the inferior alveolar neurovascular bundle to the roots of the tooth, the more likely nerve damage is to occur. Patients must have an understanding of the potential consequences of IAN damage, and

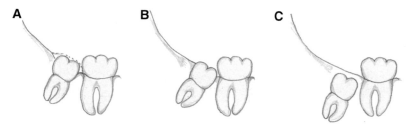

Fig. 5. Classification based on dental procedural codes. (*A*) A soft tissue impaction (D7220). (*B*) A partial bony impaction (D7230). (*C*) A full bony impaction (D7240, D7241).

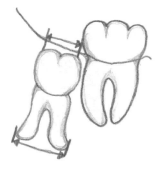

Fig. 6. If an impacted tooth—or an erupted tooth—is wider at the distal of the roots than at the crown, it must be sectioned for removal.

options such as leaving the tooth alone and coronectomy should be considered in cases in which the likelihood of IAN damage is significant [15].

The angulation classification system, the Pell and Gregory vertical relationship system (A, B, or C), and the Healthcare Common Procedure Coding System (HCPCS) coding classification also can be used for maxillary third molars. Classifying by angulation results in four types of maxillary impacted third molars (see Fig. 1A–D). Vertical maxillary impactions account for 63% of maxillary impacted third molars, whereas distoangular and mesioangular impactions account for 25% and 12%, respectively [12]. Horizontally impacted maxillary third molars are rarely encountered and, along with other angulations, account for less than 1% of impacted third molars [12]. Maxillary vertical and distoangular impactions are the easiest to remove because little bone overlies either of these presentations. In the case of mesially impacted maxillary third molars there is less access to the tooth and more bone removal is required for exposure and delivery. The bone overlying the distal aspect of this type of impaction is thicker and requires more extensive

removal. Most maxillary third molars are buccally inclined, and this position often can be confirmed by palpation. If a maxillary impacted third molar is palatally inclined, it is more difficult to remove because of more extensive bone coverage and decreased accessibility.

The Pell and Gregory A, B, C classification used in the mandibular third molars applies equally to maxillary third molars (Fig. 7A–C). Root morphology (thin, erratically curved, divided), proximity to adjacent teeth, density of overlying bone, relationship to the floor and posterior wall of the maxillary sinus, follicle size, and periodontal ligament space also play a role in determining the difficulty of the removal of a maxillary third molar impaction [12].

Bur technique

Armamentarium

An important part of third molar surgery is organization and a systematic removal strategy. The initial component of organization is having the proper instrumentation at the disposal of the surgeon at the initiation of the surgical procedure. The necessary instrumentation ideally should be contained in cassette, which allows for organization, cleaning, processing, sterilization, and transportation to the operating setting (Fig. 8). The instrumentation most commonly used for third molar removal is summarized in Box 1. Some variation in the basic set is expected because of operator preference. A properly functioning high-speed drill is a necessity. Air-driven power equipment tends to be more reliable in most cases of high-volume usage, and a Hall air drill (Linvatec, Largo, Florida) is considered one of the most popular drills.

The choice of bur is also subject to great variation. A #8 round bur is satisfactory for gross bone removal. A fissure bur lends itself better to

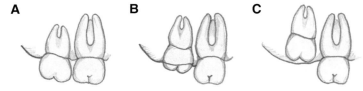

Fig. 7. Pell and Gregory classification based on the relationship to the occlusal plane applied to maxillary third molars. (*A*) Class A, in which the occlusal plane of third molar is level with that of the second molar. (*B*) Class B, in which the occlusal plane is between the occlusal plane of the second molar and its cervical line. (*C*) Class C, in which the occlusal plane of the impaction is below the cervical line of the second molar.

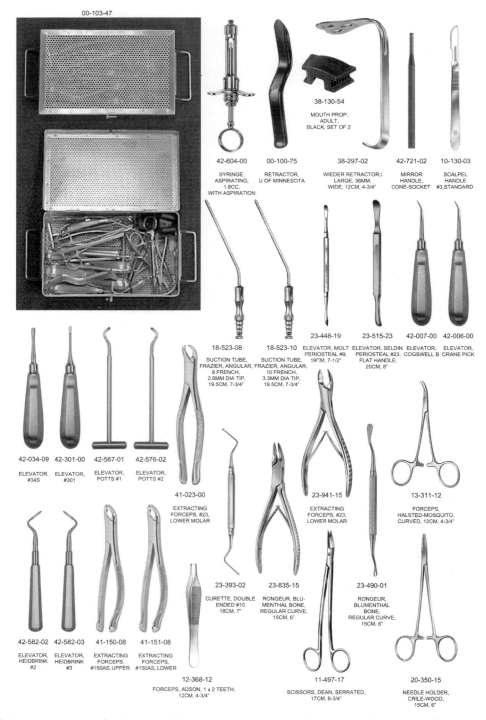

Fig. 8. A cassette system for impacted third molars. (*Courtesy of* KLS Martin LP, Jacksonville, Florida; with permission.)

Box 1. Third molar impaction/extraction tray

- Aspirating syringe
- Adult mouth prop
- Minnesota retractor
- Sweetheart retractor
- Dental mirror
- Frazier suction: 8 Fr and 10 Fr
- Scalpel handle #3
- Periosteal elevator #9
- Seldin retractor
- Elevators

#301
#34
Potts #1 & #2
Cogswell B
Crane pick
Heidbrink root tip #2 & #3

- 150 serrated forceps
- 151 serrated forceps
- Cowhorn forceps #23
- Double-ended curette
- Blumenthal end-cutting rongeur
- Side-cutting rongeurs
- Miller-Colburn bone file
- Curved mosquito hemostat
- Crile-Wood needle driver
- Dean scissors
- Adson pickup with teeth
- Martin tooth-grasping forceps

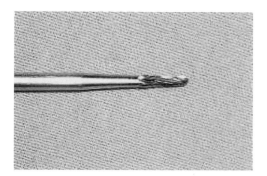

Fig. 9. Surgical bur with ideal length of 7 mm and diameter of 1.5 mm with a rounded end for gross bone removal (SS White, Lakewood NJ, #30030).

autoclaving to prevent salt build-up and clogging of the dispensing tip. A headlight, fiber optic wands, and fiber optic attachments to retractors, drills, or suction tips augment illumination provided by the standard dental or operating room lighting.

Technique

Several common steps apply to the removal of all impacted teeth. Adequate flaps must be reflected for accessibility, overlying bone must be removed for exposure, exposed teeth may be sectioned, sectioned teeth are delivered, and finally the wound must be closed. These procedures are outlined initially as they apply to third molar removal in general, and then a discussion of specific situations involving different classifications of impactions is presented. Infiltration anesthesia placed in the area overlying third molar impactions is used in addition to block anesthesia. Accessibility is a key issue in removal of impacted teeth. A full-thickness mucoperiosteal flap must be elevated to allow for visualization and placement of retractors, drilling equipment, elevators, and forceps. The lower third molar incision most commonly used is an envelope flap that extends from the mesial of the first molar to the ramus with lateral divergence of the posterior extension to avoid lingual nerve injury. An alternative incision that allows for increased exposure and less trauma to the reflected tissue is a three-cornered flap. With this flap an anterior vertical releasing incision at the distal aspect of the first or second molar is made. In either flap design the incision must be full thickness. The extent of the

trough development and tooth sectioning. There are tapered and straight fissure burs with rounded tips (eg, SS White, Lakewood, New Jersey, 1702L #30030), which combine the aforementioned tasks efficiently (Fig. 9). The fissure bur should be 1.5 mm in diameter and at least 7 mm in head length. The narrow diameter of the surgical bur allows a straight narrow sectioning of the tooth. A #301 elevator can be placed in the sectioned tooth and the tooth fractured easily. The head of the bur should be at least 7 mm in length so that an adequate depth of cut can be made before the wider shank (2.5 mm) engages the tooth.

Sterile saline is satisfactory for irrigation. It can be dispensed by syringe or automatically by devices attached to the drill and driven by a pump. If the irrigation solution is dispensed by a pump device, one should remember that all usage must be followed by a plain water flush before flap reflection should be limited to the external oblique ridge laterally. Reflecting beyond this point leads to increased dead space and more edema. The flap must be raised in a subperiosteal plane without tears. A Minnesota retractor is placed just lateral to the external oblique ridge and stabilized against the lateral surface of the mandible. The retractor should be held by a few fingers at its distal end so that it can be toed out laterally without the hand holding it blocking the vision of the operator. The need for bone removal with a drill or periosteal elevator can be established at this point.

After the need for and extent of bone removal is determined, a hand piece with adequate speed and torque is used to remove bone from the occlusal aspect of the tooth. Buccal and distal bone removal is performed down to the cervical line of the impaction. This bone removal should be in the form of a trough and should not involve the full thickness of the lateral cortical plate of the mandible. Only enough buccal cortical bone should be removed as is needed for access for elevating, sectioning, and purchase point placement. After initial bone removal the tooth should be elevated with a #301 elevator. If the entire tooth as a unit can be elevated slightly at this juncture it lessens the chance of fracturing a root tip and finding it nonmobile when an attempt to recover it proceeds. With respect to upper third molar teeth, the overlying bone in the maxilla is typically thin and usually can be removed with a Potts elevator, periosteal elevator, or chisel using hand pressure.

When sufficient access is obtained, the need for sectioning of an impacted tooth can be determined. Several key points should be mentioned regarding tooth sectioning in general. When it is determined that a tooth should be sectioned vertically (as in the case of a mesioangular impacted lower third molar), the line of sectioning generally should be determined and then moved approximately 1.5 to 2 mm more anterior than initially felt necessary. This adjustment helps prevent inadvertently sectioning the tooth too distally, which often occurs as a result of the obstructing position of the second molar. The cut through the tooth should proceed to just short of the lingual surface to protect the lingual nerve. Vertical cuts should be placed carefully so that the line of sectioning does not angle from the perpendicular. If the sectioning line varies from the perpendicular, there are cases in which the segments are wider at the bottom (in the case of the

horizontal impaction) than at the top and elevation is hindered (Fig. 10). Purchase points also can be placed at the sectioning stage. A Crane pick or Cogswell B elevator is used to elevate teeth that have purchase points placed. The purchase points should be deep enough and placed in a substantial enough portion of tooth structure so that elevation of the segment occurs rather than fracture. It should be remembered that a Cogswell B elevator has a smooth surface at the tip and is less likely to cause a fracture when used to engage the purchase point. A Crane pick is flat surfaced at the four sides of the tip and frequently causes fracturing when placed in a purchase point and force applied. When adequate bone has been removed and the tooth is sectioned into manageable segments, the tooth is delivered with elevators. The #301, Crane pick, and Cogswell B elevators serve this function well. Paired, sharp pointed elevators such as the Cryer or Winter elevators are capable of applying extreme force, and their use can be avoided if the drill is used to prepare an unimpeded pathway for delivery of the sectioned tooth. Excessive force can result in unfavorable root fracture, buccal or lingual bone loss, damage to the adjacent second molar, or even fracture of the mandible. Because impacted teeth have never sustained occlusal loading, their periodontal ligament space is wider and less tenacious, and they can be easily displaced if appropriate bone is removed and elevation forces are applied in a proper direction. Most impacted maxillary third molars are easily elevated with a #301 elevator after removal of overlying bone. A Potts elevator can

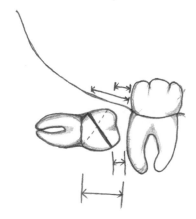

Fig. 10. Incorrectly sectioning the crown (broken line) leaves a segment that is bigger at the bottom than the top, and removal is blocked.

be used after initial elevation provides an entry point for this elevator. The Minnesota retractor or periosteal elevator always should be placed distal to the impacted maxillary third molar on final elevation so that it cannot be displaced under the flap and into the infratemporal fossa. Although not popular in the United States, a Laster retractor is an ideal retractor because it engages the tuberosity, provides excellent access, and prevents displacement of the tooth.

After the third molar is removed the socket must be debrided of all particulate bone and remaining tooth pieces. Careful irrigation under the reflected flap prevents retention of debris in this area, which can complicate healing. A rongeur, bone file, or bur can be used to smooth any sharp or rough edges of bone. All follicular fragments should be removed with a curette and mosquito hemostat. Primary closure of lower third molar sites is recommended, and although resorbable sutures suffice, some surgeons prefer nonresorbable sutures, which provide greater and longer lasting tensile stress and encourage patients to return for a postoperative visit for suture removal. The benefit of routine follow-up for third molar patients was recently questioned by Sittitavornwong and colleagues [16], however. Some surgeons are proponents of tight suturing to assist in hemostasis, whereas other surgeons believe that loose suturing leads to less edema and allows for drainage of the wound. Frequently, upper third molar sites do not require suturing because the wound is held in proper position by gravity and the surrounding soft tissues.

The specific technique for tooth sectioning varies depending on the angulation of the impacted lower third molar. In the case of the mesioangular impaction, the crown is exposed and a buccal and distal trough is created. Some mesioangular impactions can be removed simply by placing a purchase point in the mesial portion of the tooth at the cervical line and elevating with a Crane pick or a Cogswell B elevator. In other cases the distal aspect of the crown is sectioned or the distal and mesial root portions are sectioned and the distal segment of the tooth is delivered, after which the remainder of the tooth is elevated with a #301 elevator (Fig. 11A–C).

In the case of a horizontal impaction, adequate bone is removed to allow for exposure and the crown is sectioned from the roots in a vertical plane, with care taken not to allow the cut to drift distally and create a segment of crown that is larger at the bottom than at the top (see Fig. 10).

At times the crown section resists delivery, and this process can be helped by sectioning the crown segment in a longitudinal fashion (Fig. 12A). After removing the crown, the roots can be elevated with a purchase point at the superior aspect of the upper root with elevation of both roots simultaneously or the delivery of each root individually after sectioning (Fig. 12B). In all cases of sectioning the cut should be kept within the tooth structure to prevent damage to the lingual tissues or the inferior alveolar canal.

Vertically impacted mandibular third molars can be removed by several techniques depending on the depth of the impaction, the root development, and the age of the patient. When dealing with a young patient, when the bone is somewhat flexible and root development is incomplete, the tooth often can be exposed with the creation of a buccal and distal trough followed by elevation without sectioning. A purchase point is helpful in these situations (Fig. 13A). In cases in which simple elevation is not possible, the distal aspect of the crown can be sectioned and removed followed by the elevation of the remainder of the crown and root structure if the roots are fused (Fig. 13B). If the root formation is complete and divergent, it may be best to section the mesial and distal roots, with removal of the distal root followed by the mesial root (Fig. 13C). The operator should attempt to preserve as much of a "handle" as possible because dealing with small segments that have not been luxated is where most difficulty is encountered in third molar removal. A deep, vertically impacted third molar below the cervical line of the second molar and fully covered with bone can present a difficult challenge for the surgeon. In such cases the tooth should be exposed, a buccal and distal trough created, and the tooth elevated en mass with subsequent sectioning of the crown in a horizontal fashion. The roots can be elevated in one piece or sectioned and delivered as separate units with the elevation of the distal root preceding that of the mesial (Fig. 13D). It is important to maintain as much root structure as possible to serve as a "handle" for elevation.

Distoangular mandibular impactions are considered by most surgeons to be the most difficult third molar impactions to remove. The pathway of delivery for an elevated distoangular impaction is into the vertical ramus of the mandible. The goal of the technique for removal of these teeth is to create an adequate buccal and distal trough around the full crown of the tooth to a depth

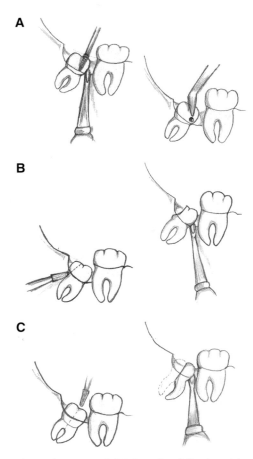

Fig. 11. Mesioangular mandibular impaction removal. (*A*) Buccal and distal trough created and tooth elevated distally with a #301 elevator or a purchase point and a Cogswell B elevator. (*B*) Distal portion of crown sectioned and removed followed by elevation of the mesial crown segment and roots. (*C*) Sectioning the roots with elevation of the distal segment followed by elevation of the mesial segment.

below the cervical line. At this point elevation of the tooth should be attempted. If some movement is obtained, the distal portion of the crown or the complete crown can be sectioned in a horizontal fashion from the roots and removed. The sectioned crown may have to be sectioned again if inadequate space is available for its removal. It is preferable in this case to section the tooth segments further as needed rather than to remove more bone. The remaining root segment along with the mesial portion of crown, in cases in which the distal portion has been eliminated as a first step, can be elevated and removed (Fig. 14A). Additional sectioning of this fragment also may be necessary to create segments that are of a size that can be removed from the bony cavity created. Additional sectioning of tooth is preferable to

additional bone removal at this point because preservation of the structural integrity of the lower jaw is maintained. If the complete crown has been removed, the remaining root segments can be dealt with as a single unit. If tooth sectioning is required, the distal root should be elevated before the mesial root (Fig. 14B).

Throughout this article, no mention or recommendation has been made by the author (SEF) for Cryer, Winter, or Cogswell A elevators. These instruments have the ability to create significant forces, and unless they are cautiously applied they can damage the teeth or bone with potential unexpected tooth, alveolar, or mandibular fracture. A sharp, pointed elevator such as a Cryer or a Winter can be useful in removing bone in the furcation that is retaining a root fragment, but

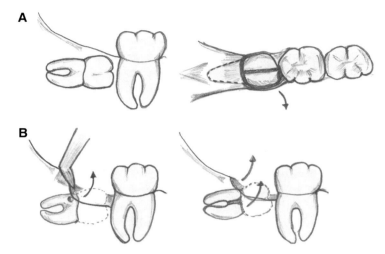

Fig. 12. Horizontal mandibular impaction removal. (*A*) The crown is sectioned from root and removed as a unit or may need to be sectioned longitudinally for removal. (*B*) Elevation of roots with a purchase point and a Cogswell B elevator. Roots may need to be sectioned into two pieces and removed separately, with upper followed by lower.

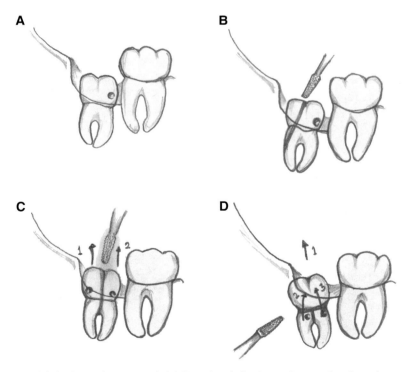

Fig. 13. Vertical mandibular impaction removal. (*A*) Buccal and distal trough created and purchase point placed and elevation with a #301 elevator or a Cogswell B elevator. (*B*) Distal crown segment sectioned and removed followed by a purchase point in the roots for elevation with a Cogswell B or a #301 elevator. (*C*) Tooth and root units split and removed distal followed by mesial with purchase points for Cogswell B and #301 elevators as required. (*D*) Crown removed horizontally and roots split for removal distal followed by mesial with purchase points for Cogswell B and #301 elevators as required.

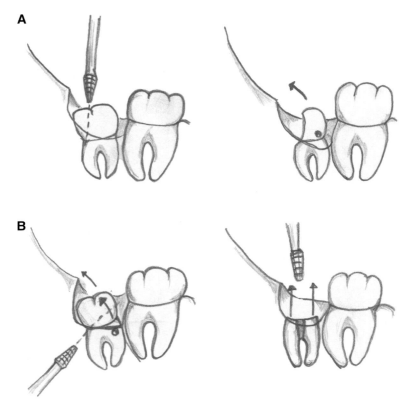

Fig. 14. Distoangular mandibular impaction removal. (*A*) Buccal and distal trough created and distal portion of crown sectioned followed by a purchase point in the mesial of the remaining tooth structure followed by elevation. (*B*) Crown sectioned horizontally and removed followed by sectioning of the remaining roots and elevation of each root independently.

a root fragment so elevated is pushed against an intact wall of bone and is more likely to fracture or defy removal than it would if removed in a mesial direction with the assistance of a well-placed purchase point as needed (Fig. 15). The use of a Cogswell A or other broad elevator between the buccal surface of the impacted tooth and the external oblique ridge to loosen or elevate a tooth or root segment is a common practice in third molar removal. This technique places the external oblique

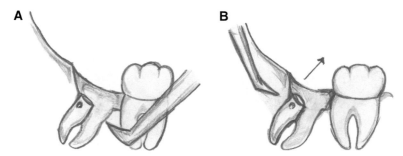

Fig. 15. (*A*) Elevation of a remaining root fragment with a Cryer- or Winter-type elevator in a distal direction removes intraseptal bone but forces the root against the intact distal socket wall, where it resists removal. (*B*) A well-placed purchase point in the distal of the root fragment allows a Cogswell B or Heidbrink elevator to guide the root mesially, where it meets no resistance to removal.

ridge, one of the buttresses of the mandible, and the lingual plate at risk for fracture. If such a fracture is unrecognized, a substantial late-presenting sequestrum or immediate lingual nerve injury is a possibility. Delicate instruments can be used to remove impacted third molars if adequate exposure, bone removal, and sectioning are performed. The author (SEF) is of the opinion that a #301 and Heidebrink root tip elevator are preferred instruments for impacted tooth removal if adequate site preparation has been completed.

In the case of maxillary third molar impactions, the envelope flap usually suffices but a vertical release at the distal aspect of the first molar frees the flap for extensive elevation if visualization of the tooth is impaired. Basic principles of flap design should be maintained, with the flap broader at the base than the apex, elevation of full-thickness mucoperiosteum, and wound closure over solid bone. A Minnesota retractor is used to retract the cheek and flap while protecting the flap and allowing visualization. If the incision is carried over the tuberosity and released in its full length, palatal retraction rarely is needed. Maxillary bone is much thinner and the underlying tooth usually can be exposed by removing this bone with a periosteal, Potts, or #301 elevator. Dense bone may require a hand piece and round bur, but this is rare. Sectioning of maxillary third molars should be avoided and considered only as a last resort because small segments can be displaced into the sinus or infratemporal fossa. The elevation of an impacted maxillary third molar is initially with a #301 elevator, and further elevation and delivery can be obtained with a Potts elevator. A Minnesota or Seldin retractor should always be placed below the cervical region of the crown before significant elevation to prevent displacement of the tooth into the infratemporal fossa. An end-cutting rongeur, a hemostat, and a Martin tooth-grasping forceps (KLS Martin, Jacksonville, Florida) (Fig. 16) are useful in the removal of teeth or fragments after adequate elevation.

Once impacted tooth removal has been completed, the remaining bony cavity can be curetted to remove any remnants of the follicle. The socket should be irrigated with saline and inspected. With respect to lower third molar teeth, if the IAN is visualized, it should be documented as intact or damaged in the operative note. If the lingual nerve is visualized, its condition also must be recorded appropriately. The upper third molar site is inspected for bony fragments, soft tissue, and the presence or absence of maxillary sinus communication. Sinus precautions should be prescribed if such an opening is recognized or suspected. The avoidance of forceful nose blowing and the prescription of antibiotics and nasal decongestants are mandatory to facilitate closure of the oro-antral communication.

Lingual split technique

The lingual split is a technique that was first described by Ward in 1956 [17]. The technique continues to be popular in the United Kingdom but has not gained wide acceptance in the United States. The technique involves the use of a chisel and mallet to remove or displace the lingual plate of bone adjacent to lower third molar teeth. A small amount of buccal bone is often removed to facilitate exposure of the crown and provide a point of application for a dental elevator. Although tooth division is usually not required, it

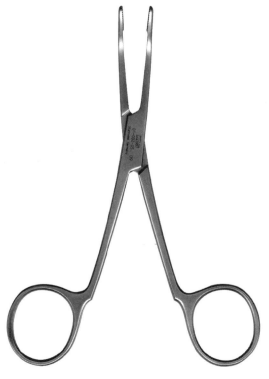

Fig. 16. Martin tooth-grasping forceps. (*Courtesy of* KLS Martin LP, Jacksonville, Florida; with permission.)

usually can be achieved with the chisel. Several minor modifications to the original technique have been reported [18,19]. Although the lingual split technique is well suited to patients receiving sedation or general anesthesia, it is generally not well suited to surgery conducted purely under local anesthesia.

The reported potential for temporary and permanent altered sensation of the lingual nerve after lingual split may be partly responsible for the technique's lack of popularity. The exact cause and timing of lingual nerve injury is not well understood and may be multifactorial. Although the original technique describes a full-thickness lingual mucoperiosteal flap, the ideal instrument for the elevation and subsequent retraction of this flap is more controversial. Most studies that evaluate lingual nerve injury are retrospective, involve small sample sizes, or are poorly controlled for multiple confounding variables and should be interpreted with some caution. Temporary lingual nerve injury has been reported to vary from 0.8% to 20%, whereas permanent injury has been reported to vary from 0% to 1% [20–23]. Although elevation of a lingual flap is an integral part of the lingual split technique, Robinson and Smith [24] recommended avoiding a lingual flap with the lingual split technique to reduce the frequency of lingual nerve injuries. One should remember, however, that lingual nerve injury is also known to occur with the standard bur technique (no lingual flap) with an incidence of 0% to 1.1%, although the duration of the altered sensation and the percentage of permanent injuries is often not stated [6,25–30]. Some surgeons advocate the use of a lingual flap in association with the bur technique to reduce the potential risk to the lingual nerve from the bur. With the use of a lingual flap, temporary and permanent lingual nerve injuries have been reported to vary from 1.6% to 8.3% and 0% to 2%, respectively [22–24, 31]. Others have found no difference in the incidence of lingual nerve injury with a bur technique regardless of whether a lingual flap is used [32]. When comparing the morbidity of lingual split to the bur technique with a lingual flap, Absi and Shepherd [33] found a greater incidence of lingual nerve injury with the bur technique, although the difference was not statistically significant. Middlehurst and colleagues [34] also found a greater incidence of nerve injury with the bur technique when comparing lingual split to the bur technique. A comprehensive review of the literature and meta-analysis by Pichler and Beirne [35] comparing lingual split, bur technique with lingual flap, and bur technique without lingual flap found an incidence of temporary nerve injury of 9.6%, 6.4%, and 0.6%, respectively. The incidence of permanent nerve injury was reported as 0.1%, 0.6%, and 0.2%, respectively. Although the lingual split technique seems to result in an increased incidence of temporary lingual nerve injury, the incidence of permanent nerve injury seems to be less than with the bur technique. It seems prudent to avoid a lingual flap with the bur technique because of the reported threefold increase in the incidence of permanent nerve injury. Differences between studies in the technique of flap elevation, choice of periosteal elevator, and retractor makes direct comparisons of morbidity difficult. It is the opinion of the author (GFB) that careful elevation of a lingual flap with an appropriate sharp periosteal elevator and placement of a suitable retractor are key factors in reducing the incidence of lingual nerve injury. Additional factors thought to influence the incidence of nerve injury include age, surgical time, perforation of the lingual plate, nerve exposure, and surgeon experience [36].

Armamentarium

Box 2 contains a list of instruments necessary for performing the split technique.

Technique

When removing a lower right third molar, the surgeon must stand on the right side of the patient. Removal of the lower left third molar

---

Box 2. Lingual split technique armamentarium

- Aspirating syringe
- Adult mouth prop
- Sweetheart retractor
- 3-mm chisel
- 5-mm chisel
- Mallet
- Scalpel #3
- Periosteal elevator #9
- Freer periosteal elevator
- Hovell's retractor
- Laster retractor
- Dental elevators (Coupland, Cryer, Warwick James)

necessitates that the surgeon stand on the left side of the patient. This is in contrast to the bur technique, which is usually performed with the surgeon standing on the same side of the patient for all third molar teeth. The surgical technique remains relatively constant regardless of the Pell and Gregory classification of the impaction. Description of the technique as it applies to a Pell and Gregory 1C impaction follows (Fig. 17). Modifications of technique for different impactions are described as needed. One should remember that occasionally a bur may be needed to facilitate tooth division or bone removal.

A rubber mouth prop is placed between the teeth on the side of the mouth contralateral to the surgery. A standard approach to anesthetize the inferior alveolar, lingual nerve, and long buccal nerve is used. An incision is made from the retromolar area to the mesial aspect of the first molar or the distal aspect of the second molar, depending on whether an envelope incision or a triangular flap is used. The latter approach involves a vertical buccal relieving incision on the distal aspect of the second molar and is preferred by the author (GFB) because it allows better retraction and improved visibility. The buccal flap is raised in a subperiosteal plane using a #9 periosteal elevator. The flap should be extended just slightly beyond the external oblique ridge to prevent excessive dead space beneath the flap. A 2-0 silk retraction suture is placed through the apex of the triangular flap. The suture should be clamped with a heavy hemostat 6 to 8 inches from the flap, which is then allowed to rest on skin of the cheek, where it serves to keep the flap retracted. Attention is then directed to raising a lingual flap, which must be done carefully to maintain a subperiosteal plane. A sharp and slightly curved periosteal elevator, such as a #9 or Freer periosteal elevator, is well suited to this procedure. The flap should be raised along a broad length before proceeding deeper. This latter approach reduces the tension placed on the lingual nerve, which adheres to the periosteum. The flap should extend from the mesial of the second molar to the lingual aspect of the anterior ramus. The inferior aspect of the pterygomandibular raphe and superior constrictor muscle together with a small portion of the mylohyoid muscle are included in this flap. One should remember that the lingual nerve enters the sublingual space by passing between the superior constrictor and mylohyoid muscles; at this location the nerve is immediately beneath the periosteum and at risk from trauma.

After lingual flap elevation, a left or right Hovell's retractor (depending on which side of the mandible is being operated) is placed beneath the flap and allowed to sit passively. The buccal flap, previously secured with the silk suture, is retracted in part from the weight of the heavy hemostat. The first finger and thumb grasp the 3-mm chisel while the second or third finger is placed on the first molar or alveolus to stabilize the instrument. The blade of the chisel is kept vertical, with the bevel facing posteriorly, and a vertical cut is made at the mesial aspect of the third molar (Fig. 18). This cut must extend from

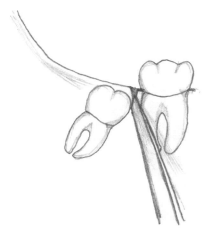

Fig. 18. A 3-mm chisel and mallet used to place a vertical cut through the lateral cortex adjacent to the mesial aspect of the crown. Inferior extent must extend sufficiently to expose an adequate amount of the tooth for application of an elevator, such as a Coupland #1 or straight Warwick James elevator.

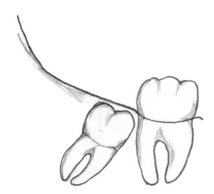

Fig. 17. Mesioangular mandibular impaction with a Pell and Gregory class 1C relationship.

the crest of the alveolar bone superiorly to a point inferiorly that allows buccal exposure of sufficient tooth to place an elevator either mesially or buccally, depending on the type of impaction present. A 5-mm chisel is then used to create a horizontal cut from the inferior aspect of the previously made vertical cut to the distobuccal aspect of the third molar (Fig. 19). The bevel should be kept facing superiorly for this osteotomy cut. The superior aspect of the buccal cortex adjacent to the third molar is delivered and exposes a portion of the third molar crown and provides a mesial or buccal point of elevation/access (Figs. 20 and 21). The most difficult and crucial aspect of the lingual split follows. The 5-mm chisel is then positioned with the edge of the blade located just posterior to the distolingual aspect of the crown of the third molar. The chisel edge should lie just lateral to the lingual cortex, and the cutting edge should be kept parallel to the sagittal plane (Fig. 22). The handle of the chisel should be approximately 45° to the horizontal. Positioning the chisel meticulously helps ensure that when the chisel is struck with the mallet, the cutting edge penetrates the superior aspect of the alveolus just inside the lingual cortex and results in displacement of the cortex lingually (Fig. 23). The anterior aspect of the fractured lingual cortex usually extends as far as the mesial of the third molar,

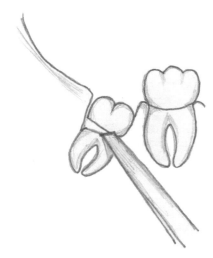

Fig. 20. The buccal ostectomy progresses in a distal direction until the complete mesiodistal width of the crown is exposed.

whereas the posterior aspect may extend up to 1 cm distally. The posterior extent of the fracture is limited by the natural bony lingual concavity behind the third molar. When the chisel blade is originally positioned for the osteotomy, the cutting edge can be rotated from parallel to the sagittal plane to shorten the posterior extent of the fracture. The inferior extent of the fracture typically involves the mylohyoid ridge (Fig. 24).

The classification of the impacted lower third molars has some influence on the applicability of the lingual split and any modifications that are needed, including the additional use of a bur for

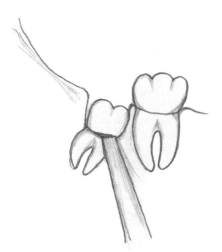

Fig. 19. A 5-mm chisel and mallet used to place a horizontal cut parallel to the cervix of the tooth. This buccal osteotomy should extend the full mesiodistal width of the crown to allow placement of a Coupland elevator between the buccal aspect of the tooth and the lateral cortex.

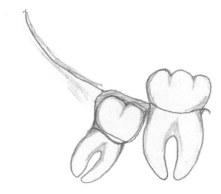

Fig. 21. After completion of the buccal osteotomies, the crown of the impacted tooth is completely visible, with good access for application of elevators.

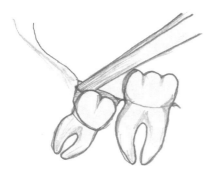

Fig. 22. The 5-mm chisel positioned just inside the lingual cortex and a single strike of the mallet is often all that is required to complete the lingual osteotomy.

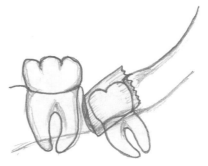

LINGUAL VIEW

Fig. 24. Viewed from the lingual aspect, the extent of the lingual cortex fracture can be seen. The inferior aspect is often attached to the mylohyoid muscle, which must be dissected free before removal of the bone.

either bone removal or tooth sectioning. With respect to the Winter classification, distoangular impactions may limit accessibility to the distolingual bone behind the tooth, making placement of the chisel for the final osteotomy difficult. This difficulty may result in a poorly controlled bone split. It may be prudent to remove the crown or distal part thereof to allow proper chisel placement. Decoronation can be completed with a bi-beveled chisel or bur, but removal of the distal portion of the crown is best completed with a bur. The author (GFB) prefers a bur for all sectioning because it provides optimal control of the sectioning. With respect to the Pell and Gregory classification, class III and C lower third molars provide the greatest challenge as they do for removal with the bur technique. Class III teeth, located almost entirely within the ramus, may

present a problem in initiating and controlling the final and most important osteotomy of the lingual plate. If bony morphology at the distal aspect allows placement of the chisel just inside the lingual cortex without facilitating propagation of the fracture up the ramus, then the procedure can continue as usual. When the bony morphology makes a controlled split unlikely, the bur technique should be used. Class C teeth that are deeply located are less of a concern and still can be managed with the lingual split technique (Fig. 25). The initial buccal exposure of the crown is readily achieved with the chisel, but when this is inadequate, a bur can be used to gain further access.

Mesioangular and horizontal impactions are also readily removed with the lingual split technique. Although the surgical procedure previously described can be applied without modification, a variable quantity of bone may overlie the most superior portion of the tooth, particularly distally. This bone should be removed before the lingual splitting osteotomy, because only then can the surgeon visualize the distolingual bone and correctly place the cutting edge of the 5-mm chisel immediately lateral to the lingual plate, resulting in a predictable lingual split (Figs. 26 and 27).

After completion of the lingual osteotomy, a dental elevator is used to displace the third molar toward the lingual space (Figs. 28–30). The need for tooth sectioning at this point is rare. When required, the sectioning is best performed with a bur after the lingual split has been completed and elevation of the tooth attempted. When sectioning is required, it may involve

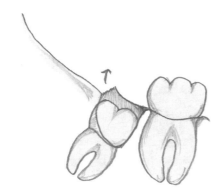

Fig. 23. The lingual cortex has been fractured lingually to provide a lingual path for removal of the impacted third molar.

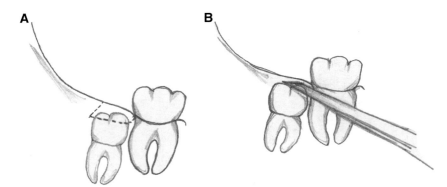

Fig. 25. (*A*) With vertical mandibular impactions (Pell and Gregory classes B and C) it is necessary to remove bone over-lying the occlusal surface of the tooth. This procedure may be completed before or after removal of the buccal cortex. (*B*) The thin overlying bone has been removed with a chisel after the buccal osteotomy was completed, which often can be completed without the mallet using hand pressure alone.

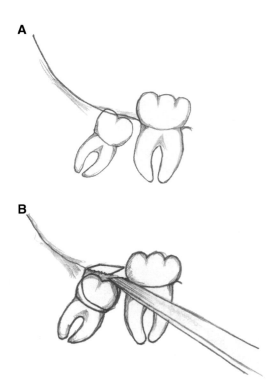

Fig. 26. (*A*) With mesioangular mandibular impactions a variable amount of overlying bone must be removed. (*B*) The overlying bone has been removed with a chisel after the buccal osteotomy has been completed. Note that the inferior extent of the buccal osteotomy does not have to extend to the inferior extent of the tooth but only as far as is needed to obtain a buccal point of application for luxation before displacing the tooth lingually.

removal of the crown or separation of individual roots. It is typically difficult to predict the need for and the type of tooth sectioning required be-cause a complete fracture of the entire lingual plate often suffices for all types of impacted third molars. It has been the author's (GFB) experience that the two most common reasons for use of a bur are (1) failure to gain adequate buccal or su-perior exposure of the unerupted tooth and (2) an unfavorable relationship between the roots and the IAN. The IAN is almost invariably located laterally with respect to the roots of the third mo-lar, however, and is less likely to be traumatized when the tooth is displaced lingually. Occasionally the preoperative radiographic appearance sug-gests an intimate relationship between the IAN and roots or clinically the angulation of the tooth seems to suggest that the roots may be lateral to the IAN. Removing the crown with a bur in com-bination with the lingual split allows the crown to be removed lingually and the roots elevated away from the IAN. One should remember that the tooth can be sectioned with a bi-beveled chisel, but the split can be less predictable and may result in tooth displacement that was not anticipated.

Once the tooth is removed, the fractured lingual cortex can be removed. Often the inferior extent of the fractured lingual plate is attached to the mylohyoid muscle, which is then removed with a periosteal elevator. The bony edges of the socket are smoothed with a rongeur and bone file. Failure to address areas of bony prominences adequately undoubtedly leads to patient discom-fort, potential future bone exposure, and possible injury to the lingual nerve. Copious irrigation

A

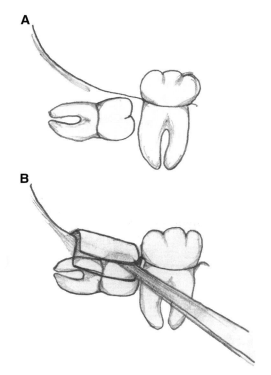

B

Fig. 27. (*A*) With horizontal impactions a significant amount of overlying bone may need to be removed. This approach occasionally may necessitate the use of a bur. (*B*) Adequate removal of buccal and occlusal bone provides a point of elevation and exposes the disto-lingual aspect of the tooth.

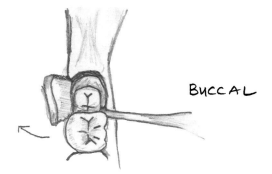

BUCCAL

Fig. 29. Occlusal view illustrates use of a Coupland elevator buccally to displace the tooth lingually.

with saline should be used to ensure that all bony splinters, which may otherwise migrate or cause infection, are removed from the wound. After the wound is inspected for hemostasis and the retraction suture removed, the wound should be closed primarily with 3-0 catgut.

Although the lingual split technique only describes removal of lower wisdom teeth, a technique using chisels for the removal of impacted maxillary third molars also is detailed for completeness. A small mouth prop is placed between the teeth on the side contralateral to the surgical procedure. Local anesthesia of the greater palatine and posterior superior alveolar nerves is obtained in

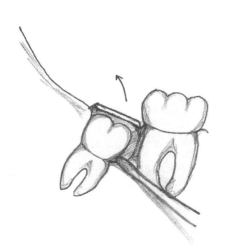

Fig. 28. Coupland #1 or straight Warwick James used to engage mesial aspect and provide initial mobility.

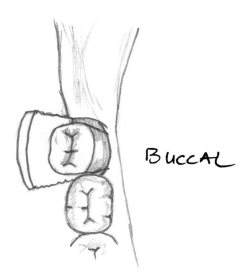

BUCCAL

Fig. 30. Occlusal view illustrates displacement of the tooth lingually for easy retrieval.

the usual manner. An oblique incision is made from a distopalatal position extending obliquely over the tuberosity toward the distobuccal aspect of the second molar before being extended into the vestibule. This oblique incision allows easy closure of the wound, often without the need for suturing. The buccal flap is then elevated to include the maxillary tuberosity. A Laster retractor can be readily positioned with the small cup-shaped tip firmly engaging the tuberosity. This retractor also protects the cheek and, by engaging the tuberosity, effectively prevents displacement of the third molar tooth into the infratemporal fossa. The retractor is held in the left hand while the surgeon stabilizes the chisel with the other hand. The chisel is held parallel to the occlusal plane and the cutting edge positioned adjacent to the distal aspect of the erupted second molar at the occlusal aspect of the alveolar process with the bevel facing toward the cheek. The assistant uses the mallet to repeatedly "tap" the chisel, which results in removal of a thin length of buccal bone from the distal second molar to the tuberosity. The chisel is positioned slightly superiorly and the process repeated. When sufficient bone has been removed, a Cryer or Warwick James elevator is positioned to engage the mesial aspect of the crown of the third molar and the tooth is displaced buccally. The soft-tissue follicle is removed carefully with a sharp curette and curved hemostat. Sharp bony areas are smoothed with rongeur or bone file before copious irrigation of the wound with saline. The wound is primarily closed with one or two 3-0 catgut sutures in the vestibular part of the incision.

Acknowledgments

The authors wish to thank Dr. Deepak Krishnan for supplying the line drawings for the article.

References

[1] Marciani RD. Third molar removal: an overview of indications, imaging, evaluation, and assessment of risk. Oral Maxillofac Surg Clin North Am 2007;19: 1–13.

[2] White RP, Shugars DA, Shafer DM, et al. Recovery after third molar surgery: clinical and health-related quality of life outcomes. J Oral Maxillofac Surg 2003; 61:535.

[3] Phillips C, White RP, Shugars DA, et al. Risk factors associated with prolonged recovery and delayed healing after third molar surgery. J Oral Maxillofac Surg 2003;61:1436.

[4] Slade GD, Foy SP, Shugars DA, et al. The impact of third molar symptoms, pain, and swelling on oral health-related quality of life. J Oral Maxillofac Surg 2004;62:1118.

[5] Foy SP, Shugars DA, Phillips C, et al. The impact of intravenous antibiotics on health related quality of life outcomes and clinical recovery after third molar surgery. J Oral Maxillofac Surg 2004;62:15.

[6] Haug RH, Perrott DH, Gonzalez, et al. The American Association of Oral and Maxillofacial Surgeons age related third molar study. J Oral Maxillofac Surg 2005;63:1106.

[7] Blakey GH, Marciani RD, Haug RH, et al. Periodontal pathology associated with asymptomatic third molars. J Oral Maxillofac Surg 2002;60:1227.

[8] White RP, Madianos PN, Offenbacher S, et al. Microbial complexes detected in the second/third molar region in patients with asymptomatic third molars. J Oral Maxillofac Surg 2002;60:1234.

[9] White RP, Offenbacher S, Phillips C, et al. Inflammatory mediators and periodontitis in patients with asymptomatic third molars. J Oral Maxillofac Surg 2002;60:1241.

[10] Shugars DA, Jacks MT, White RP, et al. Occlusal caries experience in patients with asymptomatic third molars. J Oral Maxillofac Surg 2004;62:973.

[11] Assael LA. Indications for elective therapeutic third molar removal: the evidence is in [editorial]. J Oral Maxillofac Surg 2005;63:1691.

[12] Peterson LJ. Principles of management of impacted teeth. In: Peterson LJ, Ellis E, Hupp JR, et al, editors. Contemporary oral and maxillofacial surgery. St. Louis: CV Mosby; 1988. p. 235–6.

[13] Pell GJ, Gregory GT. Report on a ten-year study of a tooth division technique for the removal of impacted teeth. Am J Orthod 1942;28:660.

[14] American Dental Association. Current dental terminology. Chicago: American Dental Association; 2005.

[15] Pogrel MA. Partial odontectomy. Oral Maxillofac Surg Clin North Am 2007;19:85–91.

[16] Sittitavornwong S, Waite PD, Holmes JD, et al. The necessity of routine clinic follow-up visits after third molar removal. J Oral Maxillofac Surg 2005;63: 1278.

[17] Ward TG. The split bone technique for removal of lower third molars. Br Dent J 1956;101:297.

[18] Davis WH, Hochwald DA, Kaminski RM. Modified distolingual splitting technique for removal of impacted mandibular third molars: Technique. Oral Surg 1983;56:2.

[19] Yeh CJ. Simplified split-bone technique for removal of impacted third molars. Int J Oral Maxillofac Surg 1995;24:348.

[20] Moss CE, Wake MJ. Lingual access for third molar surgery: a 20 year retrospective audit. Br J Oral Maxillofac Surg 1999;37:255.

[21] Rood JP. Lingual split technique: damage to inferior alveolar and lingual nerves during removal of impacted mandibular third molars. Br Dent J 1983; 154:402.

[22] Mason DA. Lingual nerve damage following lower third molar surgery. Int J Oral Maxillofac Surg 1988;17:290.

[23] Rood JP. Permanent damage to the inferior alveolar and lingual nerves during the removal of impacted mandibular third molars: comparison of two methods of bone removal. Br Dent J 1992;172:108.

[24] Robinson PP, Smith KG. Lingual nerve damage during lower third molar removal: a comparison of two surgical methods. Br Dent J 1996;180:456.

[25] Sisk AL, Hammer WB, Shelton DW, et al. Complications following removal of impacted third molars: the role of the experience of the surgeon. J Oral Maxillofac Surg 1986;44:855.

[26] Bui CH, Seldin EB, Dodson TB. Types, frequencies, and risk factors for complications after third molar extraction. J Oral Maxillofac Surg 2003;61:1379.

[27] Chiapasco M, Lorenzo D, Marrone G. Side effects and complications associated with third molar surgery. Oral Surg Oral Med Oral Pathol 1993;76:412.

[28] Goldberg B, Nemarich A, Marco W. Complications after mandibular third molar surgery: a statistical analysis of 500 consecutive procedures in private practice. J Am Dent Assoc 1985;111:277.

[29] Alling C. Dysesthesia of the lingual and inferior alveolar nerves following third molar surgery. J Oral Maxillofac Surg 1986;44:454.

[30] Bruce R, Frederickson G, Small G. Age of patients and morbidity associated with mandibular third molar surgery. J Am Dent Assoc 1980;101:240.

[31] Pogrel MA, Goldman KE. Lingual flap retraction for third molar removal. J Oral Maxillofac Surg 2004;62:1125.

[32] Chossegros L, Guyot L, Cheynet F, et al. Is lingual nerve protection necessary for lower third molar germectomy? A prospective study of 300 procedures. Int J Oral Maxillofac Surg 2002;31:620.

[33] Absi AG, Shepherd JP. A comparison of morbidity following the removal of lower third molars by the lingual split and surgical bur methods. Int J Oral Maxillofac Surg 1993;22:149.

[34] Middlehurst RJ, et al. Post-operative morbidity with mandibular third molar surgery: a comparison of two techniques. J Oral Maxillofac Surg 1988;46:474.

[35] Pichler JW, Beirne OR. Lingual flap retraction and prevention of lingual nerve damage associated with third molar surgery: a systematic review of the literature. Oral Surg Oral Med Oral Pathol Oral Radiol Endod 2001;91:395.

[36] Renton T, McGurk M. Evaluation of factors predictive of lingual nerve injury in third molar evaluation. Br J Oral Maxillofac Surg 2001;39:42.

ORAL AND
MAXILLOFACIAL
SURGERY CLINICS
of North America

ELSEVIER
SAUNDERS

Oral Maxillofacial Surg Clin N Am 19 (2007) 45–57

Office-based Anesthesia

Trevor Treasure, DDS, MD, MBA, Jeffrey Bennett, DMD*

*Department of Oral Surgery and Hospital Dentistry, Indiana University School of Dentistry,
1121 West Michigan Street, Indianapolis, IN 46202, USA*

The practice of office-based oral and maxillofacial surgery is continuously expanding and involves the management of a diverse population in regards to the surgical procedures performed within the office and the age and medical health of the patients treated within the office. Comfort, cooperation, and hemodynamic stability are critical to satisfactorily accomplishing the surgical procedure. Various anesthetic techniques are used, including local anesthesia, anxiolysis, analgesia and sedation, and general anesthesia. The topic is vast and too extensive to be discussed fully in this article. The intent of this article is to provide a discussion of some fundamental concepts that can optimize anesthetic safety and care.

Patient assessment

A careful and detailed history and physical examination should be performed on all patients undergoing office-based ambulatory anesthesia to develop an anesthesia treatment plan. Preoperative patient assessment is paramount for the safety of all ambulatory surgery patients. The American Association of Oral and Maxillofacial Surgeons (AAOMS) parameters of care document states that the anesthetist-surgeon must evaluate the patient preoperatively to determine the correct anesthetic technique and identify risk factors associated with management of that patient [1]. The medical history alone reveals up to 90% of the needed information. Laboratory examination is not typically necessary for most office-based surgery (especially third molar patients) unless dictated from the patient's underlying medical

condition. The physical examination should emphasize the cardiovascular and respiratory systems and the adequacy of the patient's airway. Airway assessment, although important to all anesthesiologists, is of special concern to oral and maxillofacial surgeons because the surgical site within the oral cavity is in close proximity to the pharynx and renders the anesthetized, nonintubated patient susceptible to airway obstruction and airway irritation. The inability to maintain a patent airway, spontaneous ventilations, and adequate oxygen saturation is a contributing factor in anesthetic morbidity and mortality.

Physical status classification

Ambulatory surgery patients should be classified according to their medical risk when undergoing a surgical procedure. This procedure is consistent with the American Society of Anesthesiologists (ASA) Physical Status Classification System, which has been in use continually since 1962. Typically, ASA physical status 1 and 2 patients can be treated safely in a dental office setting (Table 1). This represents the overwhelming majority of third molar patients. A subset of ASA 3 patients can be treated in the office provided the sedation agents benefit the patient's underlying condition through stress reduction. For example, reducing the oxygen demand on the heart through anxiolysis and analgesia for a patient with coronary artery disease benefits the patient's underlying cardiac condition. A reduction in the production of endogenous epinephrine was shown by Takemoto and colleagues [2] in a recent study after drilling bone with intravenous sedation when compared with local anesthesia alone. The ASA 4 patient should receive only local anesthesia in an office setting. Although the

---

* Corresponding author.
E-mail address: jb2@iupui.edu (J. Bennett).

Table 1
American Society of Anesthesiologists physical status classification

Classification	Description
PS-1	Normal healthy patient
PS-2	Patient with mild systemic disease
PS-3	Patient with severe systemic disease
PS-4	Patent with severe systemic disease/constant life threat
PS-5	Moribund patient
PS-6	Declared brain-dead donor patient for organ harvest

surgeon may elect not to use sedative agents on an ASA 4 patient, monitoring (eg, electrocardiography, blood pressure, pulse oximetry) should be considered.

The preanesthetic evaluation should determine if the patient is in optimal physical condition or if improvements in health can be made before extractions to reduce perioperative morbidity. Also, if warranted through the history and physical, the clinician may decide to perform the surgery in a hospital setting (Box 1) [3].

Airway assessment

Several specific components of the physical examination of the airway are pertinent to the

anesthetic management of patients, including (1) thyromental distance, (2) Mallampati classification, (3) interincisal distance, and (4) the ability to extend and flex the neck [4]. The thyromental distance is a measurement from the prominence of the thyroid cartilage to the menton with the neck in full extension. A distance less than 6 cm may predict difficulty with visualizing the larynx. The Mallampati test assesses the airway based on the ability to visualize the faucial pillars and uvula when the mouth is wide open, the tongue is maximally protruded, and the neck is extended forward. The more the base of the tongue conceals the faucial pillars and the uvula, the greater the difficulty in intubation. Normal interincisal opening should be at least 3.5 cm. Decreased opening compromises the ability to satisfactorily perform laryngoscopy and visualize the glottis [5]. The ability to flex and extend the neck is also important to facilitate alignment of the three axes of the airway to optimize direct laryngsocopy (Box 2). In a recent article, the ratio of height to thyromental distance had a higher sensitivity, higher positive predictive value, and fewer false-negative results [6]. These assessment concepts address difficulty in laryngoscopy and intubation. They are used in conjunction with the patient's history and other clinical parameters, which focus beyond the maxillofacial region to assess the patient's airway and respiratory status in regards to making an anesthetic plan for the nonintubated patient who is to have intraoral surgery (Box 3).

NPO status

Morbidity secondary to aspiration includes obstruction from particulate material and aspiration pneumonitis that depends on the quantity and acidity of the aspirate. The ASA has

---

Box 1. Specific conditions associated with significant perioperative morbidity

Congestive heart failure
Previous myocardial infarction
  (<3 months)
Critical aortic stenosis
Unstable angina
Extreme hypertension
Unstable, asthma/induction wheezing
DKA-prone diabetes
Endocrine disorders
ESRD/dialysis
Liver failure
Advanced sleep apnea

―――――

From Weaver JM. Preoperative patient assessment. In: Peterson's principles of oral and maxillofacial surgery. 2nd edition. New York: BC Decker; 2004.

Box 2. Factors associated with difficult laryngoscopy

Mallampati class 3 or 4
Neck movement ≤80°
RHTMD ≥23.5

―――――

Adapted from Krobbuaban B, Diregpoke S, Krumkeaw S, et al. The predictive value of the height ratio and thyromental distance: four predictive tests for difficult laryngoscopy. Anesth Analg 2005;101:1542.

Box 3. History and physical parameters used to assess a patient's airway and respiratory status for nonintubated sedation

History
Previous problems with anesthesia
   or sedation
Stridor, snoring, sleep apnea
Obesity
Dysmorphic facial features
Advanced rheumatoid arthritis
Spinal cord injury (eg, paraplegia)
Gastroparesis
Gastroesophageal reflux disease

Physical examination
Significant obesity
Short neck, limited extension, neck
   mass, C-spine disease
Tracheal deviation
Limited mouth opening, macroglossia,
   tonsillar hypertrophy
Vertebral disease (eg, C-spine, scoliosis,
   paraplegia/quadriplegia)

always possible. One way in which patient comfort and satisfaction may be optimized is to have the patient not have any solids past midnight and allow the patient to have clear liquids up to 2 hours before the surgery. The consumption of clear liquids up to 2 hours before administration of anesthesia has not been associated with an increase in the quantity or acidity of gastric volume. The consumption of clear liquids also may be beneficial because it can potentially minimize the risk of hypoglycemia and self-regulate the patient's hydration status, potentially minimizing adverse hemodynamic changes associated with the vasodilatory effects of various anesthetic agents. Some clinicians allow their patients to have a light meal (eg, toast and avoidance of fat-containing solids/fluids) on the morning of surgery at least 8 hours before afternoon anesthesia. Many anesthesia societies, however, still do not recommend this.

Aspiration is a significant concern in patients who do not have a protected airway. Various situations potentially increase a patient's risk of aspiration, either by their inability to protect the airway or by increasing gastric content, increasing gastric acidity, or delaying gastric emptying. Chewing gum and smoking (tobacco and cannabinoid) increase gastric volume [8]; however, the clinical significance of this is unclear. In regards to gum chewing it seems prudent to limit its use to the 2-hour restriction used for clear liquids. Smoking has numerous effects on anesthetic management beyond the potential of an increase in gastric volume, which supports the recommendation of having the patient refrain from smoking the day of surgery [9]. Pain and opioids delay gastric emptying. Gastric emptying time in obese patients is similar to nonobese patients [10]. Obese patients may be more prone to pulmonary aspirations, however, because of difficult airways and gastroesophageal reflux disease. There are other diseases in which patients may have gastroesophageal reflux disease or swallowing abnormalities that may increase the risk of aspiration (eg, cerebral palsy, hiatal hernia). Regardless of a specific organic disease, the surgeon should be respectful of a history of upper gastrointestinal symptoms and its potential to be associated with delayed gastric emptying or gastroesophageal reflux. Patients with lower gastrointestinal disease or conditions contributory to gastrointestinal stasis (eg, spinal cord injuries) also may be at increased risk. Box 4 provides a list of various medical conditions that may warrant modifications because of

published fasting guidelines to reduce the risk of pulmonary aspiration (Table 2) [7]. A minimum fasting period of 8 hours is recommended for solid food. A wakeful fasting period of this duration can be distressful to the patient and contribute to irritability, hypoglycemia, and a sensation of nausea. The easiest recommendation for avoiding these effects is to prohibit oral intake by the patient after midnight and schedule the anesthetic procedure in the morning. although it is not

Table 2
Fasting guidelines to reduce risk of pulmonary aspiration

Ingested material	Minimum fasting period (hr)
Clear liquids	2
Breast milk	4
Infant milk	6
Nonhuman milk	6
Light meal	8

Data from Practice guidelines for preoperative fasting and the use of pharmacologic agents to reduce the risk of pulmonary aspiration: application to healthy patients undergoing elective procedures: a report by the American Society of Anesthesiologist Task Force on Preoperative Fasting. Anesthesiology 1999;90:896–905.

Box 4. Common clinical conditions associated with gastroparesis

Diabetes mellitus
Addison's disease
Hypothyroidism
Hyperthyroidism
Duodenal ulcer
Systemic lupus erythematosus
Muscular dystrophy
Parkinson's disease
Depression/anxiety
Anorexia/bulimia

Data from Parrish CR. Nutrition intervention in the patients with gastroparesis. Pract Gastroenterol 2003;27:53–66.

gastroparesis [11]. Patients who have diabetes and neuropathy may exhibit delayed gastric emptying for a period up to 12 hours after a meal. Patients who have poorly controlled diabetes also may exhibit high residual gastric volumes after fasting. The consumption of clear liquids is less affected by diabetic gastroparesis. The 2-hour fast probably remains acceptable for patients who have diabetes. Patients who have Parkinson's disease may exhibit delayed gastric emptying. The severity of the motor impairment (rigor, tremor) seems to be an independent predictor of delayed gastric emptying in this disorder [12,13].

Regardless of the steps that may be taken to appropriately assess the patient and ensure that the patient has an empty stomach, there may be patients who, despite following "NPO" instructions and not having any disease or gastrointestinal symptoms that would indicate a risk for aspiration, do not truly have empty stomachs. The oral and maxillofacial surgeon always must be prepared to handle the potential of material within the airway that can result in obstruction or injury.

Smoking

Cigarette smoking has several detrimental effects on the intraoperative anesthetic management of patients. It may impact the respiratory and cardiovascular systems. From a respiratory perspective, smoking produces carbon monoxide, which elevates the carboxyhemoglobin levels 8% to 10%. There is also a leftward shift of the oxyhemoglobin dissociation curve. The net effect is less oxygen being carried by hemoglobin and

less oxygen being released to the peripheral tissues. Oxygen saturation monitoring does not detect these adverse effects. These effects may be reversed after 24 hours of smoking cessation. Smoking also impairs mucociliary clearance and promotes mucous hypersecretion, which results in the patient's airway being more irritable. Short-term discontinuation of smoking does not improve this adverse effect and actually may make the situation worse. From a cardiovascular perspective, the nicotine from tobacco smoke is an adrenergic agonist and can increase heart rate, blood pressure, and peripheral resistance. The adverse clinical adrenergic effect associated with nicotine also can be minimized by not smoking the day of surgery.

Patient maturity

Patient maturity is integral to selecting an anesthetic technique. Standard anesthetic technique used by most oral and maxillofacial surgeons entails the establishment of intravenous access and the subsequent administration of intravenous agents. Nitrous oxide or an oral benzodiazepine sometimes may be used to provide anxiolysis to make this step easier. The level of patient maturity or mental capabilities may pose a unique challenge because these patients may lack the ability to cooperate. Oral or intramuscular sedation with ketamine or inhalation of a potent anesthetic agent (eg, sevoflurane) may be necessary to establish intravenous access. A general anesthetic depth may be required to ensure the ability to satisfactorily complete the treatment.

Monitoring

Monitoring is defined as "a continuous observation of data to evaluate physiologic function." The use of monitoring permits a prompt recognition of a deprivation from normal, so corrective therapy can be implemented before morbidity ensues. An ASA closed claims case analysis concluded that routine monitoring would prevent up to 50% of patient injuries that had occurred [14]. Monitoring includes the role of the anesthetic team and assessing the respiratory, circulatory, and neurologic status.

Anesthetic team

There is a prevailing thought in medicine that human errors are inevitable and that these errors are not necessarily secondary to incompetence. An ASA closed claims analysis reported that up to 80% of anesthetic mishaps could have been prevented and were attributable to human error [14]. In various industries significant effort has been expended on trying to understand the various factors that may contribute to these errors. In medicine, the team approach has been shown to be effective in optimizing performance and minimizing these errors [15,16]. The concept of team management is consistent with that outlined in the AAOMS parameters of care and the ASA's practice guidelines for sedation and analgesia by non-anesthesiologists [17]. The anesthetic team concept is the first level of monitoring. A well-trained team ideally is an efficient organization in which safe anesthesia is administered. The concept of the anesthetic team is most important under the conditions of an emergency. The quality of the team and the interaction between its individuals are key factors affecting patient outcome. Leadership, decision making, and team coordination require practice. Mock emergency drills must be a component of the team's preparation (especially in an oral and maxillofacial surgeon's office, in which an urgent or emergent event is not an everyday event).

Respiratory monitoring

Respiratory monitoring consists of assessing the adequacy of ventilation and the maintenance of arterial oxygenation. The importance of respiratory monitoring is emphasized by the fact that in an ASA closed claims study adverse respiratory events constituted the single largest class of injury [18].

Pulse oximetry measures oxygen saturation. The monitor is sensitive and responds rapidly to sudden and potentially deleterious changes [19]. There are limitations with pulse oximetry. Foremost is the fact that the monitor does not directly measure PaO_2 (oxygenation), and in the individual receiving supplemental oxygen the initial declining changes in PaO_2 may be undetected and not reflected by changes in oxygen saturation. This fact is further impacted by the placement of the oximetry probe peripherally (on the finger). The blood must circulate from the core to the periphery before the monitor detects any abnormality. Even with this limitation, however, a decrease in arterial oxyhemoglobin desaturation should be identified before changes in skin color or hemodynamic variability. Centrally positioned probes should minimize the circulatory delay and

decrease the incidence of artifact that is associated with cold extremities. In situations in which the oximetry is not functioning secondary to cold extremities, placing a surgical glove on the hand in which the oximetry probe is placed can improve the functionality of the oximeter. Surgeons and anesthetic team members are probably familiar with the changing tone of the device that characterizes a change in oxygen saturation. To optimize any monitoring device, the alarms must be set such that the device warns when the patient is approaching conditions that can be potentially associated with adverse events. For the individual receiving supplemental oxygen, the pulse oximetry alarm should be set at 94%. This recommendation is based on an understanding of the relationship between PaO_2 and SaO_2 (defined by the oxygen-hemoglobin dissociation curve).

Anesthetic agents inherently cause respiratory depression, which manifests as decreased respiratory rate, decreased tidal volume, or airway obstruction. The AAOMS parameters of care and the ASA Task Force on Sedation and Analgesia by Non-Anesthesiologists state that "monitoring of ventilatory function reduces the risk of adverse outcomes" [17].

Several methods are used by our colleagues to monitor ventilations, including observation of chest wall excursions, observation of the reservoir bag, auscultation with a pretracheal stethoscope, and capnography. The surgeon always must be observant of the patient because nothing can replace an astute observer in detecting subtle changes. Data from any monitor must be interpreted and integrated with all of the other available information. There is a significant difference in the potential information provided between surgeon and patient provided by either auscultation with a pretracheal stethoscope or capnography compared with simply observation of chest wall excursions or the reservoir bag [20]. Although it is not conclusive whether capnography should be the standard of care for ventilatory monitoring, the authors believe that either auscultation with a pretracheal stethoscope or capnography should be used for deep sedation/general anesthesia and is consistent with the recommendation outlined in the AAOMS parameters of care document. A study published in the *Journal of Oral and Maxillofacial Surgery* in 2003 documenting anesthetic practice among oral and maxillofacial surgeons reported that approximately 40% of individuals who participated in this study used neither of these techniques for ventilatory monitoring [21].

Circulatory monitoring

In an ASA closed claims study published in the early 1990s, monitoring electrocardiogram and blood pressure had significantly less impact on preventing adverse events compared with respiratory monitoring. Anesthesia can cause hemodynamic changes, however, and it is intuitive that the blood pressure and the electrocardiogram should be monitored continuously. For the healthy individual, lead two of a three-lead electrocardiogram is used to monitor and discriminate dysrhythmias. When sedating a patient with ischemic heart disease, it may be more important to monitor lead V_5 to observe for ischemic changes. Lead V_5 has a 75% sensitivity for detecting ischemic changes compared with a 33% sensitivity for lead two. The typical monitor available in most oral and maxillofacial surgeons' offices requires some minor modifications to allow for this monitoring, which can be accomplished by relocating the LA lead to the V_5 position and setting the control to monitor lead one.

Depth of anesthetic monitoring

Current methods of assessing a patient's depth of sedation have been subjective, including observation of patient alertness, patient muscular tone, patient movement, facial expression, ptosis of the eyelids, depth of respiration, and vital signs, including respiratory rate, blood pressure, and heart rate. There are limitations to this methodology, because a patient may seem comfortable yet not be to the depth of anesthesia that the surgical-anesthetic team anticipated. Accepting that the goal of the anesthesia is to have a comfortable and cooperative patient, this limitations is not a necessarily a complication. In nonintubated patients there is not the same concern of a patient being paralyzed and awake during surgery without the ability to communicate distress. Alternatively, the lack of availability of an objective monitor to assess depth of anesthesia may result in a patient being more profoundly anesthetized than necessary. With continuous monitoring of patients and the use of anesthetic agents with predictable and relatively short duration for surgical procedures of relatively short duration, this does not necessarily result in adverse affects.

Bispectral analysis (BIS) monitoring provides an objective method of assessing the depth of sedation. The technology is an analytical analysis of the EEG that provides a number that correlates with a clinical endpoint. The BIS scale ranges from 100, which represents a completely awake individual, to 0, which represents the absence of brain activity. From a clinical perspective, a value of between 70 and 80 correlates with conscious sedation to deep sedation, a value less than 70 correlates with a high likelihood that the patient is amnestic to the procedure, and a value less than 60 correlates with an unconscious patient [22,23]. The monitoring has demonstrated benefit in reducing the quantity of anesthetic agents used and the rapidity of recovery. There are limitations, however. In situations in which either the surgical stimuli or the anesthetic state changes rapidly, the actual BIS number, which is calculated from 15 to 30 seconds of EEG data, is delayed and not "real time." For third molar surgery, which is the most common surgical and anesthetic procedure performed in an oral and maxillofacial surgeon's office, there are various periods during which the surgical stimuli is significantly altered for brief periods of time.

The surgeon must ask in which situation this monitoring is beneficial. Ketamine has seen an increase in popularity and has a certain role in office-based anesthesia. The drug differs from most anesthetic agents because it stimulates the sympathetic nervous system. The anesthetic state produced by ketamine does not correlate with the value provided by BIS. For surgeons who use a benzodiazepine and opioid technique, the drugs are usually titrated to effect at the beginning of the case. Once the anesthetic effect is achieved, the intraoperative clinical recovery from the anesthetic effect is fairly linear. Some surgeons may administer propofol or methohexital at the beginning of the case to facilitate the administration of local anesthesia but anticipate recovery from the initial bolus and intend on the anesthetic beyond that point to depend on the benzodiazepine and opioid. For these anesthetic drug combinations and techniques, the ability to incorporate BIS monitoring to assess the depth of the anesthetic should not impact the ability to care for patients safely and comfortably.

When propofol or methohexital is used as an incremental bolusing technique, the pharmacokinetics of these anesthetic agents have the potential to result in swings in anesthetic depth. For a well-trained surgeon, the knowledge that comes with experience and the artful use of a combination of drugs generally results in a comfortable and safe anesthetic. Propofol and methohexital also can be used with an infusion pump to maintain a constant therapeutic plasma drug level, ideally minimizing fluctuations in anesthetic depth. BIS monitoring may provide some guidance when a continuous infusion is used. BIS monitoring has been shown to predict the level of sedation more accurately with propofol than with midazolam [24]. Considering all of the components of third molar surgery (including the surgical site being contiguous with the airway and the airway not being intubated and the changing levels of surgical stimuli), however, the full advantages of BIS monitoring may not be appreciated fully. Alternatively, the monitoring may provide more guidance in cases in which infusions are used for surgical techniques with less intermittent stimulation, such as implant placement or bone grafts [25].

Monitoring summary

In establishing parameters and determining the usefulness of any monitor, the surgeon must consider the benefits of using a monitor, the adverse consequences of not using a monitor, and the cost of obtaining the information. A pretracheal stethoscope, including the stethoscope bell and a custom earpiece, costs less than US$100. A wireless system that can amplify the sound using an earpiece or a speaker can be assembled for less than US$250. The cost of capnography has significantly decreased. Nasal cannulas that provide oxygen and sample carbon dioxide add a few dollars' cost to each anesthetic. BIS monitoring remains more costly for the equipment and the disposable items that are required for each patient. For the usual third molar surgical procedure, the authors do not believe that the literature supports the use of BIS monitoring.

Fluid management and intravenous access

In most instances, office-based dentoalveolar surgery is of short duration and involves minimal blood loss. The need for fluid resuscitation perioperatively is not a major concern in everyday practice. A pre-existing fluid deficit occurs secondary to preoperative fasting guidelines, however. For the typical 70-kg adult patient who would be "NPO" after midnight, this results in a fluid deficit between 1L and 2 L.

To understand the concept of fluid management, the surgeon-anesthetist must understand the concept of fluid compartmentalization. Total body water exists in two major compartments. The intracellular compartment represents approximately two thirds of the total body water. The extracellular compartment represents approximately one third of the total body water and is further divided into the intravascular and extravascular compartments. The intravascular compartment represents one fourth of the extracellular space or one twelfth of the total body water. One also must understand that the intent of fluid management in office-based surgery is to rehydrate a patient as opposed to replace intraoperative fluid losses. The physiologic replacement of the deficit that results from being "NPO" can be achieved with 0.45% saline solution. The administration of an isotonic solution, such as 0.9% saline solution, provides potential advantages because it remains within the intravascular space for a longer period of time. By remaining intravascularly for a longer period of time, the fluid potentially can counter the vasodilatation secondary to the anesthetic agents. D5/W is a hypotonic solution and does not provide the physiologic benefit of 0.45% or 0.9% saline because it is rapidly distributed and equilibrated with total body water. Patients who have dentoalveolar surgery also may have impaired oral intake. Rehydration also has been shown to be beneficial in improving the quality of recovery from office-based dentoalveolar surgery/anesthesia when patients were rehydrated with 16 to 17 mL/kg of 0.9% saline solution [26].

To administer fluids, intravenous access is required. The AAOMS parameters and pathways document recommends that "intravenous access for patients receiving intravenous medications for deep sedation/anesthesia and maintenance of vascular access throughout the procedure and until the patient is no longer at risk for cardiopulmonary depression." The recommendation to maintain this vascular access throughout the procedure ensures a route for the administration of supplemental anesthetic agents and emergency medications. The use of an indwelling catheter for this intravenous access is recommended. The potential problem with hollow rigid needles is the possibility of vein lumen perforation and subsequent infiltration of fluids or drugs, which is especially problematic if the hollow needle is placed at a mobile area, such as the wrist or antecubital fossa.

Anesthetic pharmacology

Various anesthetic agents and techniques are used in office-based anesthesia to facilitate surgery and patient comfort. Amnesia, analgesia, suppression of stress response, hemodynamic stability, immobilization, sedation, and hypnosis are among the effects sought with the administration of anesthetic agents. The anesthetic agents used most commonly for third molar surgery office-based anesthesia are benzodiazepines, opioids, ultra–short-acting anesthetic agents (eg, propofol or methohexital), and ketamine. These drugs are administered in various combinations and can be administered by incremental boluses or via an infusion pump [27].

Midazolam

Midazolam is the prototype water-soluble benzodiazepine first available in 1986 in the United States. Benzodiazepines are agonist drugs at the inhibitory GABA receptor. These agents produce opening of the chloride gated channel and reduce neuronal transmission. Midazolam is contained within an aqueous solution, without propylene glycol, and causes less pain on injection. The dose for conscious sedation ranges from 0.05 to 0.15 mg/kg intravenously, typically titrated in incremental boluses. The speed of onset of midazolam is relatively slow, with a time to peak effect between 180 and 480 seconds. Respiratory depression may occur with large intravenous bolus injections of midazolam. The total dose of benzodiazepine is decreased when given together with an opioid or ultra–short-acting anesthetic agent. The effect achieved with the initial titration frequently provides an anesthetic effect for the duration of a common 30- to 45-minute procedure. For a prolonged procedure, additional incremental boluses can be administered. Alternatively, a continuous infusion of midazolam (0.25–1 µg/kg/min) can be used. Midazolam is biotransformed through oxidative-reduction (Phase 1) reactions and is susceptible to outside influences (age, cirrhosis, cytochrome p-450 inducers). Termination is largely caused by redistribution (alpha-half life) from the central nervous system, although midazolam is also rapidly cleared from the liver. The advantages of midazolam are its profound perioperative amnesia, sedation, and anxiolysis.

Opioids

Opioids may be classified as natural or synthetically derived. Opioids are primarily used to provide analgesia. If given alone, patients retain awareness and memory, and thus opioids are not true anesthetic or sedative agents. Reliable sedation cannot be achieved without producing respiratory depression. Most opioids produce a reduction in sympathetic tone. These drugs act on specific receptors within the brain and spinal cord that alter sodium channel conductance. The μ_1 receptor seems to be the major antinociception site and analgesia produced is dose dependent. Unfortunately, the μ_2 produces respiratory depression, a known untoward side effect of commonly used opioid agents. Respiratory depression is worsened by the concomitant administration of benzodiazepines or ultra–short-acting anesthetics [28]. Fentanyl is a commonly used opioid in oral and maxillofacial surgery offices. One of the advantages of fentanyl is that it does not produce increases in plasma histamine and is not associated with bronchospasm or significant vasodilatory effects on blood pressure. It is considered a short-acting agent. The accuracy of this statement depends on the actual dose and technique of administration. The dose for typical third molar surgery is in the range of 2 µg/kg. At this dose, fentanyl is clearly a short-acting agent, although the surgeon must be cognizant that the respiratory effects may outlast its analgesic effects. Fentanyl also can cause chest wall or glottic rigidity with rapid administration. The incidence of such with the relatively low dose used by oral and maxillofacial surgeons is unlikely because the speed of onset of fentanyl is relatively slow, with a time to peak effect between 180 and 300 seconds. There have been anecdotal reports of chest wall rigidity with low doses of fentanyl, however. Avoidance of administering the 100-µg fentanyl (typically contained in the 2-cc ampule) as a bolus should avoid this potential complication. An increase in the incidence of rigidity also has been reported to be associated with the rapid administration of fentanyl in combination with other agents (eg, nitrous oxide).

Historically, meperidine was the most commonly used opioid by oral and maxillofacial surgeons. Meperidine is a synthetic opioid with atropine-like effects. It was initially synthesized as an anticholinergic agent in the 1930s. Meperidine, through its vagolytic properties, can cause an increase in heart rate. It also interacts with several agents, including monoamine oxidase inhibitors and indirect-acting catecholamines (antidepressants, anti-Parkinson's drugs), to potentially cause serotonergic crisis. Remifentanil is a new class of very short-acting opioids. It is unique because the termination of its therapeutic effect depends on hydrolysis by nonspecific plasma and tissue esterases rather than redistribution from the central nervous system to the peripheral vessels. Remifentanil is most frequently used as an infusion in conjunction with incremental boluses of midazolam or a propofol infusion. In selecting an opioid, the surgeon must be familiar with the pharmacokinetics and pharmacodynamics of each agent. The reduction in sympathetic tone (which may contribute to a slowing of the heart rate) that can occur with fentanyl, especially when combined solely with midazolam is beneficial. The lack of this effect with meperidine is a disadvantage. Alternatively, remifentanil has an increased incidence of bradypnea and bradycardia and, if administered as a bolus or infused too rapidly, has an increased incidence of chest wall rigidity. At a minimum, ventilation must be monitored closely as the potential for adverse respiratory changes is potentially greater.

Propofol

Propofol is a popular agent that is used for anesthesia induction and maintenance. It is most commonly used in ambulatory office-basd oral and maxillofacial surgery to achieve a hypnotic state. It is an ideal agent because of its rapid onset, short duration of action, nonhypnotic clinical effects (eg, antiemetic, anxiolytic, amnestic, euphoria, antiseizure, central sympatholytic effect), and lack of significant adverse effects. The drug is available in a lipid-based emulsion. The drawback to this formulation is that it supports microbial growth and produces pain on injection. Three formulations are currently available in the United States, each with a different antimicrobial agent. The addition of an antimicrobial agent to the formulation resulted after several postoperative infections were associated with propofol that had extrinsically become contaminated [29]. The proprietary formulation contains ethyl-enediaminetetra-acetic acid (EDTA). There are two different generic preparations, one with sodium metabisulfite and the other with benzyl alcohol (the latter formulation having been released only recently).

There are some differences between the formulations that depend on the action of the antimicrobial agent. The antimicrobial agent sodium metabisulfite is more effective in a lower pH. The sulfite-containing formulation has a pH in the range of 4.5 to 6.4, whereas the EDTA preparation has a pH similar to the original preservative-free formulation, which is between 7 and 8.5.

There has also been discussion about a potential allergic reaction associated with the sulfite-containing propofol because sulfites are well known to cause allergic reactions. The sulfite formulation carries a warning label of this possibility, although no adverse situations have been reported in the literature.

Numerous articles have discussed the use of propofol in the oral surgical model [27,30]. It can be administered as an incremental bolus or an infusion. The bolus technique is the more common technique used by most oral and maxillofacial surgeons. Dosing for this technique is highly variable and depends on the use of preoperative sedation with benzodiazepine, opioid, or ketamine. The initial bolus may vary from as little as 20 to 40 mg of propofol to 1 to 1.5 mg/kg of propofol. An alternative to the incremental bolus technique is a continuous infusion with supplemental boluses as necessary. The intent of an infusion is to minimize the fluctuations in drug plasma concentration, which results in an improved surgical and anesthetic environment. Ideally this would result in less patient movement, improved hemodynamic stability, more rapid recovery, and less anesthetic agent use. Although many surgeons incorporate propofol into their anesthetic technique to induce a hypnotic state, it also can be used as an infusion for its sedative, anxiolytic, and amnestic properties to achieve an anesthetic state consistent with conscious sedation.

Ketamine

Ketamine was introduced in the United States in the early 1970s. Ketamine produces what is referred to as a "dissociative" anesthesia by blocking cortical awareness of external stimuli from reaching the higher centers of the brain. The dissociation occurs between the limbic system and the thalamic-cortical areas of the brain. Ketamine has several properties that are clinically advantageous. The drug achieves its dissociative anesthetic effects and its analgesic effects while maintaining protective reflexes, functional residual capacity, and spontaneous ventilations. For these reasons and the uniqueness of sedation in nonintubated patients having intraoral surgery in which the surgical site is contiguous with the airway, ketamine has had a recent resurgence in use in oral surgery. Ketamine may be incorporated into the routine regimen with a combination of benzodiazepine, opioid, or propofol. It should not be used as a sole anesthetic agent for office-based oral surgery. The purpose of its routine administration is the dissociative state that it establishes in which the patient is relatively quiescent, which creates a good working environment. Distinct from the rapid recovery with resultant movement that may be seen with either propofol or methohexital, the return of muscular activity that occurs with ketamine is slower and more robotic, which minimizes situations that may be unruly during which surgery cannot be performed. The intravenous dosing of ketamine depends on what other anesthetic agents are used. For individuals unfamiliar with the technique, however, an initial dose up to 0.5 mg/kg should be safe and efficacious [31,32]. Ketamine is also a good agent to be considered for administration in situations in which satisfactory anesthetic conditions cease to exist and the surgeon is encountering a struggling patient.

There are several potential disadvantages of ketamine. It has a central sympathomimetic effect that can result in an increase in heart rate and blood pressure. The mean increase in heart rate can approximate a 20% increase. Patients with a history of hypertension or who take various medications, such as tricyclic antidepressants, have relative contraindications to the use of ketamine. Upper airway secretions may increase secondary to the administration of ketamine. The increase in secretions could contribute to increased airway irritability and potentially laryngospasm. If this is a problem the anticholinergic agent, glycopyrrolate can be administered because it has less effect on the heart rate compared with atropine. Although most articles describe the favorable ventilatory effects of ketamine, one should remember that ketamine is an anesthetic drug that alters a patient's level of consciousness. Diligence in airway management must be observed continually because there is potential for respiratory depression and aspiration despite the favorable effects of ketamine. Ketamine also has been associated with postoperative delirium. The coadministration of midazolam should minimize the incidence of such. Finally, ketamine may prolong recovery; however, the relatively low dose of ketamine used for these techniques should not prolong it significantly.

Discharging a patient

Discharge of the patient is the sole responsibility of the anesthetist-surgeon who treated that patient. This task should not be delegated to office staff. The continuity of care by examination provides objective and subjective data to the practitioner so he or she may decide when a particular patient is stable enough to be discharged. Quantitative scoring systems are currently available to provide practical, reproducible objective criteria to decide when patients can be discharged (Box 5) [33].

Controversies in concepts in emergency management of anesthetic complications

A careful and detailed history and a physical examination and the development of an appropriate anesthetic plan may not always prevent anesthetic adverse events. The surgeon, staff, and

---

Box 5. Modified postanesthesia discharge scoring system

Vital signs
2 = within 20% of preoperative value
1 = 20–40% preoperative value
0 = 40% preoperative value

Ambulation
2 = steady gait/no dizziness
1 = with assistance
0 = none/dizziness

N/V
2 = minimal
1 = moderate
0 = severe

Pain
2 = minimal
1 = moderate
0 = severe

Surgical bleeding
2 = minimal
1 = moderate
0 = severe

Total score is 10; patients who score ≥9 are considered fit for discharge.

Adapted from Chung F. Discharge criteria: a new trend. Can J Anaesth 1995;42:1056; with permission.

office must be prepared for the most likely and most severe of these adverse events. Optimal management of anesthetic adverse events involves team management. A component of that preparation includes a surgeon's continual involvement with advanced cardiac life support courses, which must be supported by the office's ability to initiate the advanced cardiac life support protocols. More effective use of the training and emergency equipment occurs if the office has regularly scheduled mock emergency drills. Computer-based simulators for anesthetic management, emergency care, and advanced cardiac life support are also readily available from companies such as Laerdal and Anesoft. These simulators allow the doctor to demonstrate emergency situations and allow the team to be evaluated. OMSNIC also recently introduced an educational program for recognition and management of office emergencies. The AAOMS anesthesia manual also provides a succinct review of management of anesthetic emergencies and a recommendation for drugs and equipment. This section addresses some controversies.

*Should the office have succinylcholine
or a non-depolarizing neuromuscular agent?*

Succinylcholine is a synthetic, rapid-onset, and short-acting depolarizing muscle relaxant. It is most commonly stocked and used in oral and maxillofacial surgery practice for the management of laryngospasm that is refractory to positive end expiratory pressure. The initial recommended dose for a typical adult patient for management of laryngospasm ranges from 20 mg to a paralytic dose of 1 mg/kg. The onset of intravenous administered succinylcholine is approximately 30 seconds. The lower dose may terminate the laryngospasm without causing total muscle relaxation [34]. The lower dose may be ineffective in treating laryngospasm, however, and if an additional dose is required there is a potential for severe bradycardia secondary to activation of the muscarinic receptor [35]. Consideration should be given to the intravenous administration of 0.5 mg atropine before a re-bolusing of succinylcholine.

Although it provides favorable effects in terminating laryngospasm, succinylcholine has adverse effects, including muscle fasciculations and myalgia, bradycardia and hypotension, hyperkalemia and cardiac arrest, increase in intragastric pressure and risk of aspiration, prolonged paralysis (abnormal pseudocholinesterase), and triggering of

malignant hyperthermia (MH). The potential adverse effects associated with succinylcholine raise the question of its use in the management of laryngospasm. Nondepolarizing neuromuscular agents are an alternative to succinylcholine but are either slower in onset or more prolonged in duration. Rocuronium (0.6 mg/kg) has the most rapid onset of the nondepolarizing agents, with the relaxation of vocal cords occurring in 45 seconds [36]. The recovery time for the usual dose of rocuronium is approximately 30 minutes, however, which compares to a paralysis duration of approximately 5 to 10 minutes that occurs with the 1 mg/kg dose of succinylcholine. (The lower dose of succinylcholine may not cause complete muscle relaxation.) Mivacuronium is an alternative to rocuronium because duration is shorter and recovery may be seen in as short as 15 minutes. Onset is slower, however. If a nondepolarizing neuromuscular agent is to be used, the anesthetic team must be capable of providing positive pressure ventilation for 15 to 30 minutes and should consider the necessity to intubate the patient. Succinylcholine for an adult patient is—in many individuals' opinion—an appropriate agent to be used for the management of laryngospasm. In pediatric patients younger than 12 years, there must be consideration to the child not yet being diagnosed with a myopathy that could result in hyperkalemia and cardiac arrest. The US Food and Drug Administration recommends that succinylcholine be used only on indication (eg, rapid sequence induction) rather than routinely, especially in children.

Depending on the patient population treated within the office, consideration should be given to having succinylcholine and rocuronium available.

*Should dantrolene sodium be required
for offices that do not regularly use agents
that trigger malignant hyperthermia?*

The Malignant Hyperthermia Association of the United States has published the following statement: "All facilities where MH-triggering agents are administered should be prepared to treat an MH episode" [37]. The association recommends the stocking of dantrolene sodium to be prepared to treat an MH episode. In a well-written article published in current therapy in the *Journal of Oral and Maxillofacial Surgery*, the authors reviewed several state regulations pertaining to the requirement of stocking dantrolene sodium in oral surgery offices [38]. We do not necessarily agree with the conclusions of those authors that dantrolene sodium should be available but believe that dantrolene sodium should not be required to be available on-site for offices in which succinylcholine is used for emergency purposes and not regularly used. Most of our oral and maxillofacial surgery colleagues in their entire professional career have never had a situation in which succinylcholine was required to manage laryngospasm. If one's practice deviates from this frequency (although succinylcholine may be used for emergency purposes only), however, the surgeon's office should have a minimum of 12 vials of dantrolene sodium to facilitate the initial management of MH.

The patient who has MH can be administered anesthesia safely in the oral and maxillofacial surgeon's office. Deep sedation or general anesthesia can be achieved using traditional intravenous anesthetic agents. The office, however, must be prepared to manage laryngospasm with a non-depolarizing neuromuscular agent and should have dantrolene sodium.

Summary

Through its professional organization, oral and maxillofacial surgery has developed a protocol to maintain quality of anesthetic care. The protocol involves appropriate facilities, equipment, personnel, and office evaluations. This article is an extension of the principles developed from these documents.

References

[1] AAOMS parameters and pathways: clinical practice guidelines for oral and maxillofacial surgery. Version 3.0. Rosemont (IL): American Association of Oral and Maxillofacial Surgeons.

[2] Takemoto S, Nakano M, Sano K, et al. The influence of bone drilling during extraction of third molars. Anaesth.

[3] Weaver JM. Preoperative patient assessment. In: Peterson's principles of oral and maxillofacial surgery. 2nd edition. New York: BC Decker; 2004.

[4] Mallampati SR, Gatt SP, Gugino LD, et al. A clinical sign to predict difficult tracheal intubation: a prospective study. Can Anaesth Soc J 1985;32:429.

[5] Wilson ME, Spiegelhalter D, Roberson JA, et al. Predicting difficult intubation. Br J Anaesth 1988; 61:211.

[6] Krobbuaban B, Diregpoke S, Krumkeaw S, et al. The predictive value of the height ratio and thyromental distance: four predictive tests for difficult laryngoscopy. Anesth Analg 2005;101:1542.

[7] ASA Task Force on Preoperative Fasting. Anesthesiology 1999;90:896.

[8] Soreide E, Veel T, Holst-Larsen H, et al. The effects of chewing gum on gastric content before induction of anesthesia. Anesth Analg 1995;80:985–9.

[9] Schumacher A, Vagts DA, Noldge-Schomburg GF. Smoking and preoperative fasting: are there evidence-based guidelines? Anaesthesiol Reanim 2003; 28:88–96.

[10] Maltby JR, Pytka S, Watson NC, et al. Drinking 300 mL of clear fluid volume and pH in fasting and non-fasting obese patients. Can J Anaesth 2004;51:111–5.

[11] Parrish CR. Nutrition intervention in the patient with gastroparesis. Pract Gastroenterol 2003;27:53–66.

[12] Goetze O, Nikodem AB, Weizcoek J, et al. Predictors of gastric emptying in Parkinson's disease. Neurogastroenterol Motil 2006;18:369–75.

[13] Jellish WS, Kartha V, Fluder E, et al. Effect of metoclopramide on gastric fluid volumes in diabetic patients who have fasted before elective surgery. Anesthesiology 2005;102:904–9.

[14] Cooper JB, Newbower RS, Kitz RJ. An analysis of major errors and equipment failure in anesthesia: considerations for prevention and detection. Anesthesiology 1984;60:34.

[15] Sexton J, Thomas E, Helmreich R. Error, stress, and teamwork in medicine and aviation: cross-sectional surveys. BMJ 2000;320:745.

[16] Bellomo R, Goldsmith D, Uchino S, et al. Prospective controlled trial of effect of medical emergency team on postoperative morbidity and mortality rates. Crit Care Med 2004;32:916–21.

[17] American Society of Anesthesiologists Task Force on Sedation and Analgesia by Non-Anesthesiologists. Practice guidelines for sedation and analgesia by non-anesthesiologists. Anesthesiology 1996;82:459.

[18] Bhananker SM, Posner KL, Cheney FW, et al. Injury and liability associated with monitored anesthesia care: a closed claims analysis. Anesthesiology 2006;104:228–34.

[19] Cote CJ, Goldstein EA, Cote MA, et al. A single-blind study of pulse oximetry in children. Anesthesiology 1988;68:181.

[20] Bennett J, Petersen T, Burleson JA. Capnography and ventilatory assessment during ambulatory dentoalveolar surgery. J Oral Maxillofac Surg 1997;55: 921–5.

[21] Perrott DH, Yuen JP, Andresen RV, et al. Office-based ambulatory anesthesia: outcomes of clinical practice or oral and maxillofacial surgeons. J Oral Maxillofac Surg 2003;61:983.

[22] Sandler NA, Hodges J, Sabino M. Assessment of recovery in patients undergoing intravenous conscious sedation using bispectral analysis. J Oral Maxilllofac Surg 2001;59:603–11.

[23] Sandler NA, Sparks BS. The use of bispectral analysis in patients undergoing intravenous sedation for third molar extractions. J Oral Maxillofac Surg 2000;58:364–8.

[24] Ibrahim A, Taraday JK, Kharasch ED. Bispectral index monitoring during sedation with sevoflurane, midazolam, and propofol. Anesthesiology 2001;95: 1151–9.

[25] Sandler NA. Additional clinical observations using bispectral analysis. Anesth Prog 2000;47:84.

[26] Bennett J, McDonald T, Lieblich S, et al. Perioperative rehydration in ambulatory anesthesia for dentoalveolar surgery. Oral Surg Oral Med Oral Pathol Oral Radiol Endod 1999;88:279–84.

[27] Bennett J, Shafer DM, Efaw D, et al. Incremental bolus versus a continuous infusion of propofol for deep sedation/general anesthesia during dentoalveolar surgery. J Oral Maxillofac Surg 1998; 56:1049.

[28] Bailey PL, Pace NL, Ashburn MA, et al. Frequent hypoxemia and apnea after sedation with midazolam and fentanyl. Anesthesiology 1990;73:826.

[29] Bennett SN, McNeil MM, Bland LA, et al. Postoperative infections traced to contamination of an intravenous anesthetic, propofol. N Engl J Med 1995; 333:147–54.

[30] Candelario LM, Smith RK. Propofol infusion technique for outpatient general anesthesia techqniue. J Oral Maxillofac Surg 1995;53:124.

[31] Blankstein KC. Low dose intravenous ketamine: an effective adjunct to conventional deep conscious sedation. J Oral Maxillofac Surg 2006;64:691.

[32] Mehrabi M, Perciaccante V, Roser S. Efficacy and adverse effect of ketamine in outpatient oral and maxillofacial surgery adult patients. J Oral Maxillofac Surg 2005;63:74.

[33] Chung F. Discharge criteria: a new trend. Can J Anaesth 1995;42:1056–8.

[34] Chung DC, Rowbottom SJ. A very small dose of suxamethonium relieves laryngospasm. Anesthesiology 1993;48:229.

[35] Stoelting RK, Peterson C. Heart rate slowing and junctional rhythm following intravenous succinylcholine with and without intramuscular atropine preanesthetic medication. Anesth Analg 1975;54: 705.

[36] Laurin EG, Sakles JC, Panacek EA, et al. A comparison of succinylcholine and rocuronium for rapid-sequence intubation of emergency department patients. Acad Emerg Med 2000;7:1362.

[37] Malignant Hyperthermia Association of the United States. All facilities where MH-triggering agents are administered should be prepared to treat an MH episode. Available at: http://www.mhaus.org/index.cfm/fuseaction/OnlineBrochures.Display/BrochurePK/ABD1DA74-4433-48F3-A4C7902B67F6FCFB.cfm. Accessed.

[38] Collins CP, Beirne OR. Concepts in the prevention and management of malignant hyperthermia. J Oral Maxillofac Surg 2003;61:1340.

ORAL AND
MAXILLOFACIAL
SURGERY CLINICS
of North America

ELSEVIER
SAUNDERS

Management of the Impacted Canine and Second Molar

Pamela L. Alberto, DMD*

*Department of Oral and Maxillofacial Surgery, University of Medicine and Dentistry of New Jersey,
New Jersey Dental School, Newark, NJ, USA*

Impacted canine and impacted second molars are problems frequently encountered by oral and maxillofacial surgeons. Success in management along with the development of a satisfactory treatment plan requires a team effort with input from the orthodontist, general dentist, and surgeon. Although the overall prevalence in the population is low, the impacted maxillary canine is second only to the impacted mandibular third molar in its frequency. We find that the population incidence is only between 1.7% and 2.2% [1]. Second molar impaction incidence is even less, at approximately 0.4%. The condition is twice as common in girls (1%–2%) as in boys (0.5%) [2]. Impacted canines are found palatally in 85% of cases, with labial position in 15% of cases. Having both conditions is rare, as seen in Fig. 1. For the purpose of this article, we discuss the management of the impacted canine and second molar.

Impacted maxillary cuspid

Etiology

Calcification of the maxillary canine starts at age 1 and is completed in 5 to 6 years. It remains high in the maxilla above the root of the lateral incisor until the crown is calcified. The maxillary cuspid erupts along the distal aspect of the lateral incisor, which closes the physiologic diastema present between the maxillary central incisors. The maxillary canine travels almost 22 mm during the time of eruption. It first moves in a palatal direction then buccally. The maxillary canine should erupt before 13.9 years for girls and before 14.6 years for boys [3]. The origin of impaction is unclear but most likely is multifactorial. Because the maxillary canine has the longest path of eruption in the permanent dentition, alteration in position of the central and lateral incisor may be a factor. Arch length discrepancy and space deficiency may result in the canine becoming labially impacted. Studies have shown a higher incidence of palatally impacted canines in cases with missing lateral or peg-shaped incisors. Failure of the primary canine to resorb may cause palatal movement of the permanent canine, although Thilendar and Jakobsson [3] considered failure of resorption of the primary canine to be a consequence rather than a cause of impaction. A genetic predisposition has been shown in some studies. Pirinen and colleagues [4] found that palatally impacted canines are genetic and related to incisor-premolar hypodontia and preshaped lateral incisors.

Other possible causes are trauma to the anterior maxilla at an early age, pathologic lesions, odontomas, supernumerary teeth, and ankylosis. There is also a higher incidence of impacted maxillary canine after alveolar bone grafting in patients who have a cleft [5].

Localization

Localization of the maxillary canine is a key factor in the comprehensive assessment of the impacted canine. The position of the impacted canine is important when deciding management options for patients. Localization requires inspection, palpation, and radiographic evaluation. The

* 171 Woodport Road, Sparta, NJ 07871.
E-mail address: alberto@umdnj.edu

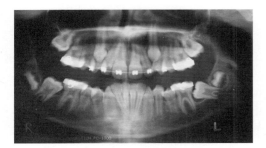

Fig. 1. Impacted maxillary and mandibular canines with an impacted mandibular second molar.

position of the lateral incisor can give a clue to the canine position. The crown of the lateral root may be proclined if the canine is lying labial to the lateral incisor. Occasionally the impacted canine can be palpated on the labial or palatal aspect. The surgeon can take a series of periapical radiographs along with a panoramic radiograph to locate its position. When taking the series of periapical radiographs, the cone head is shifted horizontally so Clark's Rule can be used to discern the buccal or lingual position of the canine. I find that 45° to 60° anterior occlusal views provide the shifting necessary to localize the position of the canine. Cephalometric radiographs and CT scans are also useful in determining location of the impacted canine, but they are more costly. If you need to extract the over-retained primary canine, the resorption pattern on the root provides a clue to localization of the crown of the impacted cuspid. Sometimes you can feel the crown when giving your infiltration anesthesia on the buccal and palatal mucosa.

Treatment options

After the patient undergoes a clinical and radiographic evaluation, a comprehensive treatment plan can be developed. An informed consent with discussion of treatment options and alternatives is important to avoid misunderstanding or legal problems. Treatment options include (1) no treatment except monitoring, (2) interceptive removal of primary canine, (3) surgical removal of the impacted canine, (4) surgical exposure with orthodontic alignment, and (5) autotransplantation of the canine.

No treatment with periodic radiographic evaluation

No treatment is recommended if the canine is in good position and without contact with the lateral incisor and first premolar. If there is no evidence of pathology or root resorption of the adjacent teeth or the patient refuses treatment, the patient can be monitored periodically. If the impacted canine is severely displaced and remote from the anterior teeth and is difficult to remove or expose, a decision can be made to monitor the patient radiographically. Ferguson and Pitt [6] surveyed all the UK consultant orthodontists to assess their opinion on management of the impacted maxillary canine in patients for whom no orthodontic treatment is planned. They found that most orthodontists were in favor of removal of the impacted canine, with a significant minority suggesting the conservative approach of radiographic monitoring.

Interceptive removal of primary canine

Extraction of the primary canine is recommend if the patient is between 10 and 13 years, the maxillary canine is not palpable, and localization confirms a palatal position (Fig. 2). If the canine position does not improve over a 12-month period, alternative treatment is indicated. Radiographic evaluation should be at 6-month intervals. Figs. 3 and 4 shows a case in which the primary canine was removed and it erupted within 6 months.

Surgical removal and prosthetic replacement

Surgical extraction of the impacted canine is indicated when there is poor position for orthodontic alignment, there is early evidence of resorption of adjacent teeth, the patient is too old for exposure, and the degree of displacement does

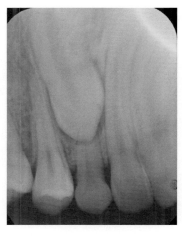

Fig. 2. Extraction of primary canine to facilitate eruption of impacted canine.

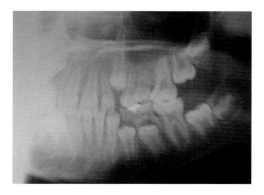

Fig. 3. Extraction of primary canine.

not allow for surgical reposition or transplantation. The treatment of choice for replacement of the canine is a dental implant. Sometimes orthodontic treatment is needed to provide enough space for implant placement.

Flap design. Flap design is dictated by the location of the impacted canine. If the impacted canine is located buccally, a gingival crest incision can be made in the gingival sulcus. If the impacted canine is high, the incision can be made horizontally above the papillae. Vestibular incisions made at the level of the mucogingival junction should be made only when the impacted canine is above the root apices. If the impacted canine is palatal, a palatal incision placed in the gingival sulcus can be performed. Palatal incisions placed between the gingival crest and palatal vault should be avoided, because trauma to the greater palatine artery could occur. Occasionally, the impacted canine can be positioned transversely in the alveolus,

which would require mucoperiosteal flaps on the palatal and labial sides.

Surgical removal. Bone generally is removed using a #8 round bur with copious amounts of irrigation. A 301 straight elevator is used to achieve movement of the tooth. Usually sectioning of the crown from the root is required for removal. Then the remaining portion of the root can be removed. If an implant is planned, a bone graft in the extraction site for ridge preservation is recommended.

Surgical exposure

Surgical exposure is the conventional treatment for impacted canines. There are three methods used for surgical exposure and orthodontic alignment [7]: (1) open surgical exposure, (2) surgical exposure with packing and delayed bonding of the orthodontic bracket, and (3) surgical exposure and bonding of orthodontic bracket intraoperatively. If the canine has correct inclination, the open surgical exposure is the treatment of choice. Excision of the gingiva over the canine with bone removal is sufficient to allow eruption of the canine [8].

If surgical exposure with orthodontic alignment has been chosen as the method of treatment, three surgical approaches can be used. The replacement flap technique replaces the mucoperiosteal flap over the exposed canine after the bracket and chain are applied. A disadvantage of this technique is that bonding can fail and re-exposure is necessary. The excisional exposure removes the mucosa overlying the crown of the impacted canine. The apically repositioned flap is used to preserve the attached gingiva (Fig. 5). Vermette and colleagues [9] found that apically repositioned flaps resulted in more aesthetic

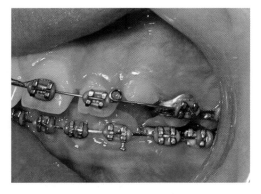

Fig. 4. Normal eruption of canine after primary canine extraction.

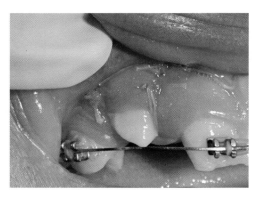

Fig. 5. Apically repositioned flap.

problems than the replacement flap technique. The goal is to choose a technique that exposes the canine within a zone of keratinized mucosa without involvement of the cemento-enamel junction. This approach minimizes potential periodontal complications after orthodontic alignment.

If the inclination of the canine to the midline is more than 45° then the prognosis for alignment worsens. The closer the impacted canine is to the midline the worse the prognosis.

Application of orthodontic traction devices. Many different devices can be applied to the crown of an impacted canine, including a wire, pins, crown formers, and orthodontic brackets. Wires placed around the crowns of an impacted canine can injure the root of the tooth. Screwing pins into the enamel of the canine can damage the crown of the tooth. Crown formers placed or cemented over the crown of the impacted tooth were popular for many years; however, they acted as a foreign body and caused inflammation and eruption. The device of choice is an orthodontic bracket or gold mesh disk with a gold chain bonded onto the canine crown surface (Fig. 6).

Two types of bonding agents can be used. One is a two-part, self-cure bonding agent and the other is a light cure bonding agent. The advantage of the light cure materials is that most can work in a partially wet field (Fig. 7). The gold mesh disks also work better than the orthodontic brackets or buttons with the light cure bonding agent because the curing light can get at all the bonding agent through the mesh. It cannot cure the bonding agent under the bracket.

The tooth surface must be acid etched for 30 seconds and then irrigated. Success improves with hemostasis. Once hemostasis is achieved, the

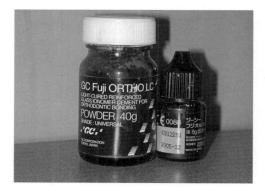

Fig. 7. Light cure bonding material used in partially wet field.

primer can be placed on the tooth. The bonding agent is placed on the bracket and pressed firmly against the enamel surface of the tooth. If it is a light cure material, it should be light cured for 20 to 40 seconds (Fig. 8). The chain that is attached to the bracket is then ligated to the patient's arch wire (Fig. 9). The orthodontist should activate the appliance within a week. The vector of force used to move the canine can be changed to move the canine away from the incisor roots and then move it vertically and buccally.

Autotransplantation of the canine

Selected maxillary impacted canines can be autotransplanted. This technique may be recommended when the degree of malposition is too great to make successful orthodontic alignment or interceptive measures have failed. This procedure surgically is more difficult than orthodontic repositioning. Moss [10] found that in adults the success of autotransplantation of the impacted canine is poor. Canine transplantation should be

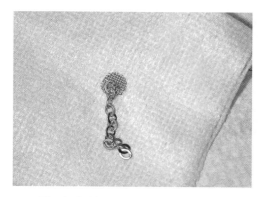

Fig. 6. Gold mesh disk with gold chain.

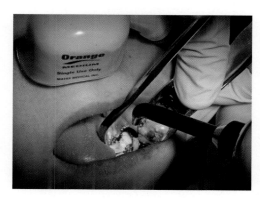

Fig. 8. Light cure for 20 to 30 seconds.

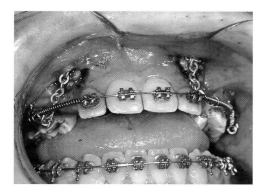

Fig. 9. Brackets ligated to arch wire.

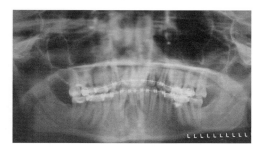

Fig. 11. Mandibular canines in occlusion after 6 months of treatment.

planned as early as possible when the root is 50% to 75% formed. The transplanted tooth must be held in place for 2 to 3 months with an orthodontic appliance. If endodontic treatment is necessary, it should be performed when the immobilization device is removed.

Impacted mandibular canines

The mandibular canine is ten times less frequently impacted than the maxillary canine (Figs.10 and 11). The mandibular cuspid has the largest root of all the teeth. The mandibular canine follicle forms at the level of the inferior border of the mandible. Because the body of the mandible is labial to the alveolus, it may explain the fact that most impacted mandibular canines are labially impacted. Similar to maxillary canines, mandibular canines are three times more common in female patients than male patients.

A treatment plan can be developed once the impacted mandibular canine is localized and assessment of potential damage to adjacent teeth and involvement of the mental nerve is made. Localization is achieved in the same manner as impacted maxillary canines.

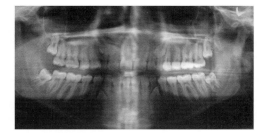

Fig. 10. Impacted mandibular canines (pretreatment).

Impacted mandibular canines are usually vertically impacted close to the labial surface. Occasionally, they can be located beneath the apices of the mandibular incisor. They are rarely found in a horizontal position.

Management of impacted mandibular canines includes the following treatment options:

- No treatment with clinical and radiographic observation
- Surgical extraction
- Surgical exposure to aid eruption
- Surgical exposure with orthodontic guidance
- Transplantation

No treatment, only observation

If the impacted mandibular canine is below the apices of the teeth and without pathology, it can be observed periodically.

Surgical extraction

If the impacted mandibular canine is not in an upright position, extraction should be considered. Surgical extraction is accomplished by using a labial or lingual mucoperiosteal flap with possible releasing incisions. The removal of bone over the crown is achieved with a round bur. The tooth can be luxated and removed with an elevator. If this approach is unsuccessful, the crown is sectioned and the crown and root are removed. If the mandibular canine is lingual, the extraction is more difficult because of poor access.

Surgical exposure to aid eruption

If the mandibular canine impaction is caused by an overlying impediment, the impediment can be removed surgically. Then a bony pathway for eruption can be created.

Surgical exposure with orthodontic guidance

Four types of incisions can be used for exposing the impacted mandibular canine [11]: (1) the labial gingival crevice incision, (2) alternative labial gingival crevice incision, (3) free mucosal incision, and (4) lingual gingival crevice incision. The labial gingival crevice incision is an incision in the gingival sulcus from the right first premolar to the left first premolar that preserves the interdental papilla. A vertical releasing incision can be used if additional access is required. The alternative labial gingival crevice incision is a horizontal incision made at the base of the interdental papilla. Closure of the incision is more difficult. A vertical releasing incision also can be used if more access is required. The free mucosal incision is used when the impacted mandibular canine is located at the level of the apices of the incisors or lingual to them. The incision is placed a few millimeters away from the mucogingival junction in the nonkeratinized mucosa horizontally. The incision should remain anterior to the mental foramen to avoid the mental neurovascular bundle.

If the impacted maxillary canine is lingual to the incisors, the lingual gingival crevice incision should be used. The incision is made in the lingual gingival sulcus from the mandibular right first premolar to the mandibular left first premolar. The incision should be extended to provide adequate access. Releasing incisions should not be used. If the lingually impacted mandibular canine is below the level of the apices of the incisors, an extraoral approach may be necessary.

Transplantation

Transplantation of the mandibular canine can be successful if the apex of its root has not closed. The canine can be transplanted to its correct position in the dental arch or even to a different site. The difficulty is in removing the tooth without damaging the root surface or apical end. The canine must be firmly immobilized for at least 2 months. The endodontic procedure can be performed on this tooth after immobilization.

Complications and side effects

Complications and side effects with the treatment of the impacted maxillary and mandibular canine are as follows:

Ecchymosis of the upper lip or lower lip and chin

Infection
Paresthesia
Damage to adjacent structures
Noneruption
Loss of soft tissue flap/dehiscence
Lack of attached gingiva
Devitalization of the pulp
Pain

Ecchymosis of the upper or lower lip and chin

An ecchymotic area can occur in the soft tissue if proper hemostasis is not achieved before closure. It also can occur if the patient is on aspirin or herbal medications that increase bleeding time.

Infection

Any surgical wound can develop an infection even with the best aseptic technique. With maxillary impacted canines, infections can develop in the lip, canine space, or palate. With the mandibular impacted canine, infections can develop in the lip, submental space, and sublingual space. Treatment consists of antibiotics and incision and drainage.

Paresthesia

When the mandibular impacted canine's location is near the neurovascular bundle, paresthesia may be a sequela of surgery. If the maxillary canine is impacted palatally, the nasopalatine nerve may be affected, although it rarely presents a problem for the patient. If the mandibular canine is located near the mental foramen, the patient may have a paresthesia of the lower lip and chin. Surgery performed midsymphysis may produce altered sensation in the incisors and gingiva.

Damage to adjacent structures

If the impacted canines are near the roots of neighboring teeth, the surgery could damage the impacted tooth or adjacent teeth. Displacement of a root into the maxillary sinus or nasal cavity can occur during surgical removal. Rarely, an oral antral or oral nasal fistula can follow surgical removal in the maxilla.

Noneruption

When eruption does not occur, the treatment plan should be reviewed. The most common causes of noneruption are ankylosis, inadequate interdental space, and gingival scarring.

Loss of soft tissue flap

Loss of the soft tissue flap is the result of interruption of its blood supply or infection. Flaps that are thin may have compromised blood supply. Allowing the acid etch material to come into contact with the tissues can comprise the vitality of the flap.

Lack of attached gingiva

Poor quality gingival mucosa may occur with exposure of labially impacted maxillary canine. The flap technique must preserve keratinized tissue. A connective tissue graft can be placed to correct this problem.

Devitalization of the pulp

If symptoms of pulpitis develop when the impacted canine is being orthodontically moved, the orthodontic therapy should be stopped and the canine should be evaluated for possible endodontic treatment. If adjacent teeth develop symptoms of pulpitis, endodontic therapy should be considered. This complication is rare in young individuals.

Pain

Patients experience some pain with any surgical procedure; however, there is slightly more postoperative pain from maxillary impacted canine surgery than surgery of other impacted teeth. Postoperative management during the first 24 hours should include nonsteroidal anti-inflammatory drugs and long-acting local anesthesia. Narcotic agents occasionally are necessary to relieve postoperative pain.

Impacted second molars

The impaction of the second molar is a rare complication in tooth eruption. The incidence is approximately 0.03% to as high as 3%, depending on the study. It usually occurs unilaterally more commonly than bilaterally and occurs slightly more often in men. It is more common in the mandible than maxilla. The management of impacted second molars has been a challenge for orthodontists and oral and maxillofacial surgeons. The impacted second molar is usually recognized when orthodontic treatment is complete and the roots are fully formed. Proper alignment of the second molar into the dental arch in an angle Class I position is an integral part of completing orthodontic therapy.

Management of impacted second molars requires a team approach with the orthodontist, oral and maxillofacial surgeon, and general dentist.

Etiology

There are multiple causes for impacted second molars. When the deciduous second molar is lost, the first permanent molar must move forward to accommodate the eruption of the second molar. If this does not occur, the eruption of the second molar is compromised, which can lead to tipping. If the developing third molar infringes in the space required for the second molar to erupt, mesial tipping occurs. Ill-fitting first molar bands are an iatrogenic cause of the mesial impacted second molar.

Localization

A panoramic radiograph is optimal to evaluate the position of the impacted second molar. Periapical radiographs are also useful, especially using Clark's Rule, because it tells you if the clinical crown is tilted buccally or lingually.

Treatment options

The degree of impaction and location of the second molar determine if a surgical, orthodontic, or combined approach is used. Impacted second molars must be treated. Not treating this condition and simply observing is not an option. Lack of treatment causes periodontal disease with bone loss and decay of the first and second molars. The following treatment options can be used to treat the impacted second molar.

  Surgical extraction of the impacted second molar
  Surgical extraction of the impacted third molar and surgical uprighting of the second molar
  Transplantation of the third molar into the impacted second molar site
  Extraction of the impacted second and third molar and placement of a dental implant

Surgical extraction of the impacted second molar

One treatment option involves extracting the impacted second molar and allowing the third molar to migrate forward into the second molar position. The eruption of third molar is not predictable. Often, the third molar only migrates anteriorly slightly and then tips into the second molar space, which predisposes the second molar to periodontal problems because of its malposition. Second molar extraction is contraindicated when the third molars are smaller or poorly formed, are in a horizontal position, are in the maxillary sinus, or have a severe space deficiency. It is important to make patients aware that the eruption of the third molar is not predictable and the third molar may need extraction.

Surgical uprighting of the second molar with extraction of third molar

Usually the decision to upright the impacted second molar is made by the orthodontist. The patient is referred to an oral and maxillofacial surgeon to discuss this combined orthodontic and surgical approach. This treatment plan may not be successful if the second molar root has two-thirds root formation.

After appropriate local anesthetic blocks, an incision is made along the cervical areas of the first molar along the external oblique ridge. A full-thickness mucoperiosteal flap is elevated. A round bur is used to expose the crown of the impacted second molar and third molar. It is important to avoid exposing the cemento-enamel junction and root surface, which increases the chance of periodontal defects and external resorption. The third molar is sectioned and elevated from its bone socket. Using a 301 elevator, the second molar is gently elevated. If the second molar can be elevated into proper position, then an orthodontic appliance is not required. Sometimes stabilizing the uprighted second molar can be a problem. If it is unable to self-stabilize in the surrounding bone, an orthodontic bonding material is used to bond the second molar to the first molar (Figs.12 and 13). This procedure is not required with maxillary

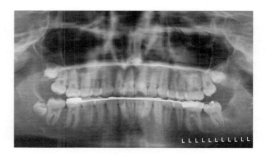

Fig. 13. Impacted second molar surgically uprighted with removal of third molar.

impacted second molars. Luxation of the tooth stimulates eruption. In Fig. 14, the second molar was exposed and luxated. Within 6 months, the tooth erupted. After eruption, the third molar was removed (Fig. 15).

Often an orthodontic appliance must be placed to upright the second molar. Going and Rayes-Lois [12] reported on a technique in which the second molar is bracketed with a band that contains a buccal tube. A heavy gauge nickel titanium arch wire is threaded through the tube. The arch wire is ligated to the two premolars and canine and helps to upright the second molar. Other appliances can be used. For example, segmental springs and nickel titanium coil springs have been successful in uprighting second molars [13,14]. With the advent of endosteal implants, microimplants that can be placed in the alveolar bone have been developed. They are used as an anchorage device. A 2-week healing period is necessary before elastics are placed. This method is used especially when trying to upright lingually tipped lower second molars and buccally tipped upper second molars [15]. Brass wire also can be used as

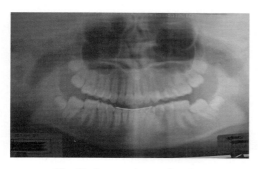

Fig. 12. Impacted second molar.

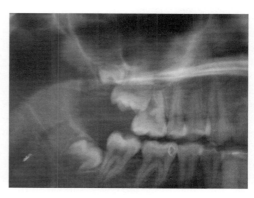

Fig. 14. Impacted maxillary second molar.

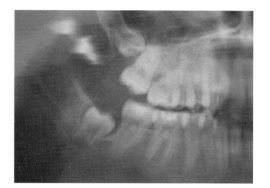

Fig. 15. Impacted second molar erupts into position after luxation.

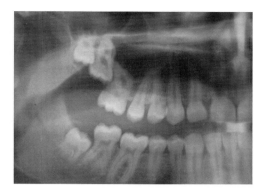

Fig. 16. Impacted maxillary second molar fully developed.

a separator when placed below and above the contact point between the first molar and impacted second molar. The wire can be tightened incrementally to upright the second molar. This technique is used infrequently because it causes pain, swelling, and future periodontal problems.

Transplantation of the third molar into the second molar position

This treatment plan can be performed if the third molar has two-thirds root development. The impacted second molar must be extracted, and then the third molar is extracted as atraumatically as possible. The third molar is wedged within the second molar socket. If the tooth is not stabilized between the buccal and lingual cortices, bonding material should be placed to keep it in its proper position without mobility. Transplantation is only possible in select cases. Once firm mobilization has occurred, endodontics must be performed.

Extraction of the impacted second and third molars with dental implants

If the age of the patient and the stage of root development are limiting factors, one should consider extracting the impacted second and third molars as an option. This treatment plan should be considered with older patients who have complete root formation (Fig. 16). With the excellent success rates of dental implants, replacing the second molar with dental implants is a predictable option.

Risk factors and complications

As with any surgical procedure, complications are possible, and they should be discussed with the patient before surgery [16]. Risk factors and complications include (1) loss of teeth, (2) root injury, (3) external resorption, and (4) periodontal defects.

Loss of teeth

Loss of the first, second, and third molars is possible if treatment is not performed. These teeth are usually lost to decay and acute periodontal disease.

Root injury

Uprighting a second molar can cause root injury and loss of vitality. If the second molar roots are fully formed there is a greater chance of root fracture or injury. Treating the impacted second molar when the roots are two-thirds developed prevents this complication.

External resorption

If the cemento-enamel junction or root surface is exposed or damaged when surgically exposing the second molar, external resorption is possible. Care should be taken to stay above the cemento-enamel junction and not expose the root surface.

Periodontal defects

When the second molar is surgically uprighted, a bone defect remains distal to the first molar. If bone fill is absent in that area, a periodontal defect develops, which gives the second molar a poor prognosis. Treating the periodontal defect with guided tissue regeneration techniques—using a bone graft and barrier—is an option.

Summary

Management of impacted canine and second molars can be difficult but rewarding. Treatment planning in these cases should be multidisciplinary. The decision to correct these impacted teeth surgically usually is made by orthodontists. Patients then seek consultation with an oral and maxillofacial surgeon concerning the treatment plan.

Usually the risk-to-benefit ratio favors the preservation of the impacted canine and second molar. Generally the recommendation is surgical exposure of the impacted canine with orthodontic alignment into the arch. It is also recommended to upright the second molar and remove the impacted third molar. Close follow-up by the orthodontist and surgeon is important to the success of these procedures. Preserving these teeth is an important orthodontic standard of care. It is important that treatment be based on an appropriate diagnosis and consultation with the orthodontist.

References

[1] Thilander B, Myrberg N. The prevalence of malocclusion in Swedish school children. Scand J Dent Res 1973;81:12–20.

[2] Dasch SF, Harrell FV. A survey of 3874 routine full mouth radiographs. Oral Surg Oral Med Oral Pathol 1961;14:1165–309.

[3] Thilander B, Jakobsson SO. Local factors in impaction of maxillary canines. Acta Odontol Scand 1968; 26:145–68.

[4] Piriren S, Arte S, Apajalahti S. Palatal displacement of canine is genetic and related to gongenital absence of teeth. J Dent Res 1998;75:1742–6.

[5] Semb G, Schwartz O. The impacted tooth in patients with alveolar clefts. In: Anderson JO, editor. Textbook and color atlas of tooth impactions. Copenhagen (Denmark): Munksgaard; 1997. p. 331–48.

[6] Ferguson JW, Pitt SKJ. Management of unerupted maxillary canines where no orthodontic treatment is planned: a survey of UK consultant opinion. J Orthod 2004;31(1):28–33.

[7] McSterry PF. The assessment of and treatment options for the buried maxillary canine. Dent Update 1996;23:7–10.

[8] Ferguson JW, Pervizi F. Eruption of palatal canine following surgical exposure: a review of outcomes in a series of consecutively treated cases. Br J Orthod 1997;24(3):203–7.

[9] Vermette ME, Kokich VG, Kennedy DB. Uncovering labially impacted teeth: apically positioned flap and closed eruption techniques. Angle Orthod 1995;65:23–32.

[10] Moss JP. The unerupted canine. Dent Pract 1972;22: 241–8.

[11] Alling C, Helfrick J, Alling R. Impacted teeth. Philadelphia: WB Saunders; 1993. p. 215–6.

[12] Going R Jr, Rayes-Lois D. Surgical exposure and bracketing techniques for uprighting impacted mandibular second molars. J Oral Maxillofac Surg 1999; 57:209–11.

[13] Majourau A, Norton L. Uprighting impacted second molar with segmental springs. Am J Orthod Dentofacial Orthop 1995;107:235–8.

[14] McAboy CP, Gruvent J, et al. Surgical uprighting and repositioning of severely impacted second molar. J Am Dent Assoc 2003;134:1459–62.

[15] Park J, Kwon O, Sung J, et al. Uprighting second molars with microimplant anchorage. J Clin Orthod 2004;38(2):100–3.

[16] Felsenfeld A, Aghaloo T. Surgical exposure of impacted teeth. Oral Maxillofacial Surg Clin N Am 2002;14:187–99.

ELSEVIER
SAUNDERS

Oral Maxillofacial Surg Clin N Am 19 (2007) 69–84

ORAL AND
MAXILLOFACIAL
SURGERY CLINICS
of North America

Therapeutic Agents in Perioperative Third Molar Surgical Procedures

Mehran Mehrabi, DMD, MD, John M. Allen, DMD,
Steven M. Roser, DMD, MD*

*Division of Oral and Maxillofacial Surgery, Emory University School of Medicine,
1365-B Clifton Road NE, Suite 2300-B, Atlanta, GA 30322, USA*

Surgical extraction of third molars is one of the most common of all surgical procedures. The outcome of third molar surgery includes pain, trismus, edema, nausea, infection, and alveolar osteitis. The intent of this article is to provide a literature review and analysis of the various chemotherapeutic agents used to control, minimize, or eliminate these outcomes. Unfortunately, comparison of the published studies represents a tremendous challenge because of the variability in parameters and methods used for each study. A trend does exist among many of the current researchers, who realize that randomized, controlled, evidence-based research rather than personal experience is necessary to develop appropriate guidelines for using chemotherapeutic agents.

Antibiotic therapy

An ideal prophylactic chemotherapeutic agent reduces the risk of predictive postoperative complications without producing serious side effects or disrupting the surgical procedure. The objective is to make the surgical experience as pleasant as possible. Fewer perioperative adverse effects translate into fewer complaints, fewer postoperative visits, and fewer dissatisfied patients.

Therapeutic agents can be administered prophylactically or empirically. A therapeutic agent provided before a surgical procedure represents prophylactic therapy. A therapeutic agent provided after surgical treatment represents empiric therapy.

Taking into consideration all surgery, the administration of antibiotics is based on wound classification. Wounds may be classified as clean, clean-contaminated, contaminated, or dirty. A clean wound is one that is free of infection or inflammation and does not involve the alimentary, biliary, respiratory, or genitourinary tracts. The risk of developing infection in a clean wound is less than 2%. Common oral surgical procedures that can be considered clean wounds include temporomandibular joint surgery and facial cosmetic surgery. Antibiotic prophylaxis is considered optional for clean wounds. A clean-contaminated wound is associated with elective procedures that involve the alimentary, biliary, respiratory, and genitourinary tracts. Examples in oral surgery include orthognathic procedures and dental extractions. The risk of infection for a clean-contaminated wound is 10%. A contaminated wound includes inflamed tissue, such as cellulitis, whereas a dirty wound consists of spillage of pus into the surgical site. An example of a clean-contaminated wound in oral and maxillofacial surgery is a maxillary fracture in a patient with active maxillary sinusitis. A dirty wound would be a mandibular fracture through an impacted third molar that is draining pus. Infection rates within contaminated and dirty wounds are 20% and 40%, respectively [1]. Antibiotic prophylaxis is recommended for clean-contaminated, contaminated, and dirty wounds [2].

Postoperative wound infection is a costly problem in the United States. When considering all surgical procedures, the prevalence is estimated at 1 million patients annually. This translates into a $1.5 billion increase in health care costs. The

---

* Corresponding author.
E-mail address: sroser@emory.edu (S.M. Roser).

average hospital stay is increased by 1 week and the cost by 20% [3,4]. Although third molar surgeries are generally performed in an ambulatory setting and do not commonly result in serious nosocomial infections, efforts focused on preventing excessive recovery periods caused by wound complications and infection are undoubtedly beneficial economically. With the cost of antibiotic therapy being small compared with extended hospital stay, antibiotic therapy should be provided to all patients who have increased susceptibility to infection.

Surgical patients who undergo extraction of third molars are generally healthy and are not likely to develop postoperative infection. Factors that increase the risk of postoperative infection in any surgical procedure includes diabetes, alcoholic cirrhosis, end-stage renal disease, corticosteroid use, old age, obesity (more with abdominal surgery), malnutrition, recent surgery, massive transfusion, preoperative comorbid disease, and American Society of Anesthesiologists (ASA) patient classification 3,4, and 5 [2]. There are few controversies in the literature regarding prophylaxis or empiric antibiotic therapy in patients with comorbid diseases. It is also generally accepted that patients who require extraction of third molars who are afflicted with any systemic disease that compromises the immune defense system against bacterial infection (eg, neutropenia, leukopenia, splenectomy, leukemia, α-γ-globulinemia, or myeloproliferative disease), are candidates for antibiotic therapy before and after surgery. There is little controversy regarding preoperative antibiotic treatment of active infection, such as fascial space infection or dentoalveolar abscess, when involved with symptomatic third molars. Finally, until proven otherwise, one must continue to prescribe antibiotics for patients susceptible to subacute bacterial endocarditis and prosthetic joint infections [5,6]. One also must realize that the wound classification in these patients for treatment of asymptomatic third molars is clean-contaminated.

Postoperative infection is a subject with a remarkable history. From the 1600s to 1800s, infections were so common that "laudable pus," warmth, and redness were considered desirable features. The first decline in postoperative infection is attributed to Semmelweis and Holmes (1800s), who adapted a hand-washing technique, and Lister (1867), who used carbolic acid spray in the operating room. Steam autoclaving of instruments was introduced by Koch, and standard operating room attire consisting of a cap, gown,

and sterile rubber gloves was introduced by Halstead in late 1880s [7]. These antiseptic principles were not taken to heart until the early twentieth century, however, when a dramatic drop was observed in postoperative infection rates.

Early in the antibiotic era, prophylactic antibiotic therapy was thought to be associated with higher rates of infection and resistance. This belief was disproved, however, in a study by Burke, who administered penicillin to guinea pigs before and after inoculation of surgical wounds with *Staphylococcus aureus*. He found that guinea pigs treated with penicillin shortly before and after inoculation with the bacteria did not develop infection, whereas guinea pigs not treated with penicillin and those treated as late as 3 hours after inoculation developed severe infections [8]. This finding demonstrated that the timing of prophylactic antibiotic therapy has great significance.

Ultimately, the timing of a surgical incision should correspond with the peak systemic concentration of an administered antibiotic. In a randomized prospective trial of 2847 patients who underwent elective clean and clean-contaminated procedures, the time of prophylactic antibiotic administration and the prevalence of postoperative infection were evaluated. The patients were divided into four groups. One group, which consisted of 369 patients, received antibiotic therapy 2 to 24 hours before surgery. The second group, which consisted of 1708 patients, received antibiotics within 2 hours of the surgery. The third group, which consisted of 282 patients, received antibiotics perioperatively. The fourth group, which consisted of 488 patients, received antibiotics postoperatively. The incidence of postoperative infection was reported to be 6.7%, 1.0%, 2.4%, and 5.8%, respectively, among the four groups [9]. Note that the highest rate occurred within the group that received antibiotic therapy more than 3 hours before surgery. It has been determined that the ideal timing for prophylactic antibiotic therapy is 30 minutes to 2 hours before surgery, with additional coverage extending for one to two half-lives of the prescribed antibiotics for the length of the operation [2].

Proper administration of antibiotic prophylaxis requires evaluation of various factors, including the type of procedure performed, organisms involved, and the choice of the antibiotic, including dosing and administration intervals [10]. The ultimate goal of therapy consists of targeting the antibiotic to a specific organism. Identification of the organisms involved in infections at third molar sites has been difficult. In evaluating the microbial complex in the third molar region, White and colleagues [11] identified a higher prevalence of anaerobic bacteria, including *Prevotella intermedia*, *Campylobacter rectus*, *Bacteriodes forsythus*, *Bacteriodes gingivalis*, and *Treponema denticola*. This anaerobic population was found to exist even when periodontal probing depths were normal. Peterson [10] found that aerobic streptococci were the most commonly found organisms present in infected postoperative third molar wounds. This variety in the microbial population creates difficulty choosing appropriate preoperative antibiotic therapy. Peterson also recommended the use of a bactericidal over a bacteriostatic agent when the antibiotic was to be used prophylactically and recommended penicillin as the ideal agent. The dose of the antibiotic should be twice the therapeutic dose and should be given no more than 2 hours before surgery [10].

The overall complication rate after third molar surgery has been estimated to be between 2.6% and 30.9% [12–26]. In a multicenter study, Haug and colleagues [16] noted that the rate of postoperative infection after extraction of third molars ranges from 0.5% to 27%. More recent studies performed by Haug and colleagues and Bui and Dodson [18] show a narrower range, with average infection rates of less than 1% regardless of antibiotic administration. Table 1 summarizes the findings of 13 recent studies reporting the incidence of infection after third molar surgery. From these reports it seems that the risk of postoperative infection increases with mandibular extractions [20,24], increased time of surgery [25], decreased operator experience [24], and increased surgical complexity [20]. There is little evidence to support prophylactic antibiotic treatment of maxillary teeth or erupted mandibular teeth. There may be some benefit to prophylactic treatment of impacted mandibular third molars, however. Chiapasco and Marrone [20] reported an infection rate of 2.4% after the removal of 1000 full bony impacted mandibular third molars. They found that the only factor to increase the incidence of operative infection among the patients was age older than 34 years.

The variability of postoperative infection rates as seen in Table 1 supports routinely prescribing and not prescribing antibiotics as part of the removal of asymptomatic impacted third molars, thus making it surgeon's preference. For the actively infected patient and the compromised patient who is medically more susceptible to infection, prophylactic antibiotics are indicated and should be administered 1 to 2 hours before the removal of the impacted third molars. The presence of anaerobic bacteria at the third molar site without any evidence of periodontal disease supports the use of prophylactic antibiotics in all cases of impacted third molar removal, including for patients who have a history of at least one episode of pericoronitis. A cogent argument against the routine use of prophylactic antibiotics in third molar removal is the possibility of the emergence of antibiotic-resistant organisms. To date, however, this occurrence has not been documented in cases of third molar removal.

There may be evidence that antibiotics in addition to chlorhexidine and copious wound irrigation may prevent alveolar osteitis [27]. The primary cause of alveolar osteitis is unknown. It has been theorized that fibrinolytic activity by oral bacteria may be responsible for this postoperative complication. Alveolar osteitis does occur more frequently in women and smokers and in patients who use birth control pills [28,29]. Metronidazole and tetracycline may be effective in preventing alveolar osteitis [30–32]. Because metronidazole is commonly used against anaerobic organisms, it is possible that alveolar osteitis is caused by oral anaerobic organisms [33].

Steroids

Extraction of third molars, as with any surgical procedure or traumatic insult, results in an intense inflammatory response that consists of edema, erythema, pain, warmth, and loss of function. This response occurs because of mediator release of cytokines, prostaglandins, and histamine from leukocytes, endothelial cells, and mast cells. The increase in osmotic pressure within injured tissue and leakage from capillaries are responsible for the expansion of tissue that occurs with edema [7,34]. Maximal edema after surgical extraction of third molars was found to occur 24 to 48 and 48 to 72 hours after surgery by Laskin [35] and Peterson [36], respectively. Corticosteroids have been shown to reduce post–third molar extraction edema [37].

The anti-inflammatory effect of corticosteroids was first identified by Hench and colleagues [38] during treatment of rheumatoid arthritis. Steroids act by interfering with capillary vasodilation, leukocyte migration, phagocytosis, cytokine production, and prostaglandin inhibition. The inhibition of capillary vasodilation prevents leakage of intravascular fluid into the interstitial space. The leakage

Table 1
Incidence of infection after third molar surgery

Author	Year of publication	Patients	Teeth	Antibiotic therapy	Risk of infection per tooth (%)
Haug [16]	2005	3760	8333	No ABT	0.5
Figueirdo [17]	2005	772	958	Some with ABT	1.5
Bui [18]	2003	583	1597	Post ABT in 94%, Pre ABT 1%	0.5
Piecuch [19]	1995	2134	6713	No ABT	14.8
				Systemic ABT	10.3
				Systemic and topical tetracycline	2.4
Chiapasco [20]	1993	614	500 maxillary 1000 mandibular	Group I 18–24 no ABT, mandible	1.2
				Group II 25–34 no ABT, mandible	1.2
				Group III <34 no ABT, mandible	2.2
Happonen [21]	1990	136		Penicillin	13
				Tinadazole	10
				Placebo	11
Michell and Morris [23]	1987	91	172	Total (with topical ABT)	11
Mitchell [22]	1986	50	89	Tinadazole group/ mandible	8
				Placebo group/ mandible	44
Sisk [24]	1986	208	1202	Faculty	1
				Resident	3.7
Osborne [13]	1985	9574	16127	No ABT	3.4
Goldberg [15]	1985	302	500	Total infection 1 infection with ABT 20 infections with no ABT	4.2
Curran [26]	1974	68	133	With ABT	7.8
				Without ABT	8.7
Nordenram [25]	1973	144		Placebo vs. Nebacetin cone	20.3

Abbreviation: ABT, antibiotic therapy.

of fluid and leukocytes results in irritation of free nerve endings and the release of pain mediators, including prostaglandin and substance P. Corticosteroids act to prevent inflammation and reduce pain at the site of insult. The extent of the reduction in inflammation by steroids is dose dependent and increases as the plasma concentration in proximity to insult reaches the therapeutic range [39].

Corticosteroids have numerous effects on the body. They are involved in fluid and electrolyte balance, metabolism of fats, carbohydrates, proteins, and purines, and homeostasis of the nervous, renal, and cardiovascular systems [40]. Continuous daily administration of corticosteroids for 1 month results in suppression of the adrenal glands and internal corticosteroid production. Patients require a doubling of their daily steroid dose on the day of the surgery, followed by a gradual tapering postoperatively back to the original daily dose matching surgical stress.

Adrenal insufficiency may occur up to 1 year after cessation of steroid therapy. Even if these patients have discontinued their steroid therapy for up to 1 year, a tapering dose of steroids may be required for surgery. Intraoperative adrenal insufficiency most commonly presents as hypotension that is resistant to fluid treatment but responds to steroid therapy. When adrenal insufficiency is suspected preoperatively, a cortisol stimulation test can be performed. An initial cortisol level is obtained, adrenocorticotropic hormone is injected, and a cortisol level is measured in 1 hour. If the cortisol level does not increase in the second measurement, a diagnosis of primary adrenal insufficiency can be made [41].

The relative potency of all steroid preparations is determined by direct comparison to cortisol. Prednisone has been determined to be 3.5 times as potent as cortisol, with prednisolone being 4 times as potent and methylprednisolone and triamcinolone being 5 times as potent. Betamethasone and dexamethasone are 25 and 30 times as potent as cortisol [42,43]. Prednisone, prednisolone, and methylprednisolone are short acting; triamcinolone is intermediate acting; betamethasone and dexamethasone are long-acting steroid preparations. The body's daily production of cortisol is 15 to 30 mg, which may increase up to 300 mg during a stressful event [40,44–46]. The normal concentration of cortisol in a healthy patient is 13 µg/dL (range 7–22), which may increase to 50 to 73 µg/dL in patients with septic shock [39]. To achieve the ideal result in preventing inflammation and pain, a high preoperative dose of steroids should be administered (above physiologic level), followed by a short-term, tapering postoperative regimen [43,47,48].

The bioavailability of glucocorticosteroids after oral administration is remarkably high and may provide effects that parallel intravenous administration. Gastrointestinal side effects, however, are known to occur from oral intake. Steroids given orally 3 to 4 hours before surgery lessen gastrointestinal upset; in an outpatient environment, however, patient compliance may not always be optimal in regards to the timing of administration. The most common steroid regimens used for orthognathic surgery are intravenous methylprednisolone, 125 mg, or decadron, 8–12 mg, given just before surgery. The most common postoperative medication prescribed is the methylprednisolone "dose pak," which is taken as a tapered dose [7,34,49–51]. It is important to note that a tapered dose of steroids after third molar surgery is prescribed not to compensate for adrenal suppression but rather to correlate with the decline in surgical stress in the 72-hour postoperative period.

The adverse effects of prolonged steroid administration are extensive. They include poor wound healing, hypertension, electrolyte abnormalities, psychosis, euphoria, osteoporosis, hyperglycemia, central obesity, abdominal striae, thin skin, glaucoma, myopathy, amenorrhea, hirsutism, acne, and adrenal insufficiency [52,53]. Although recognition of infection may be masked by steroid administration (elevated white blood cell count), patients are not more susceptible to infection after a short duration of steroids [7]. Absolute contraindications to steroid therapy include active herpes, active tuberculosis, acute psychosis, and acute glaucoma. Relative contraindications include diabetes mellitus, hypertension, osteoporosis, peptic ulcer disease, infection, renal disease, Cushing's syndrome, and diverticulitis [40,54].

In summary, short-term corticosteroid therapy may be used to decrease postoperative edema and discomfort associated with third molar extractions, with few to any side effects [40,53,55]. Short-term steroid therapy is not associated with the development of adrenal crisis [39,56–58]. There is considerable debate regarding the ideal preparation and dosage of corticosteroids for third molar extractions. Table 2 summarizes 20 third molar studies listing the dosage of steroids, route of administration, and effect on edema, pain, and trismus.

Analgesics

Postoperative pain may be reduced by various interventions (Table 3). Preoperative systemic analgesics reduce pain by inhibition of central and peripheral pain receptors. The peripheral nerves can be blocked by local anesthesia or chemotherapeutic agents [59]. Stimulation of pain receptors after an insult may result in primary or secondary hyperalgia [60,61]. Primary hyperalgia occurs at the site of the assault immediately after injury and is induced by heat or mechanical stimulation. Secondary hyperalgia occurs within the surrounding tissue adjacent to the area of primary assault [62]. Prophylactic analgesic therapy is intended to inhibit the effects of the surgery on the surrounding tissue.

Postoperative analgesics can affect either central or peripheral pain receptors. Common centrally acting analgesics include opioid narcotics. Peripherally acting analgesics primarily inhibit

Table 2
Third molar surgery and steroids

Study	Agent	Route	Dose	Edema	Pain	Trismus
Ross [53]	Hydrocortisone	PO	40 mg, BID/QID, pre (1) and postop (2)	SR	CR	CR
Ware [88]	Dexamethasone	PO	1 mg, TID, pre (1) and post (2)	CR	NR	CR
Mead [89]	Triamcinolone	PO	4 mg, TID, pre (1) and post (1)	SR	SR	SR
Linenberg [90]	Dexamethasone	PO	1mg, TID, pre (1) and post (1)	CR	NR	CR
Nathanson [91]	Betamethasone	PO	0.6 mg, QID, post (4)	CR	CR	CR
Hooley [54]	Betamethasone	PO	1.2 mg, QID, pre (2), post (1)	CR	CR	CR
Caci [92]	Prednisolone	PO	10 mg, Q4–6H, post (4)	CR	SR	SR
Byested [93]	Methylprednisolone	PO	12 mg, BID–TID, pre (1), post (2)	CR	CR	CR
Messer [94]	Dexamethasone	IM	4 mg, x1, post (1)	CR	CR	CR
Ediby [95]	Dexamethasone	IM	4 mg, QD, pre (1), post (1)	NSR	NSR	NSR
Skejelbred [96]	Betamethasone	IM	9 mg, x1, post (1)	SR	SR	SR
Skejelbred [97]	Betamethasone	IM	9 mg, x1, pre (1)	SR	SR	SR
El Hag [98]	Dexamethasone	IM	10 mg, x2, pre (1), post (1)	NR	SR	SR
Pederson [99]	Dexamethasone	IM	4 mg, x1, pre (1)	SR	CR	SR
Huffman [51]	Dexamethasone	IV	4 mg, x1, pre (1)	SR	CR	CR
Huffman [51]	Methylprednisolone	IV	125 mg, x1, pre (1)	SR	CR	CR
Sisk [50]	Methylprednisolone	IV	125 mg, x1, pre (1)	SR	CR	CR
Beirne [34]	Methylprednisolone	IV	125 mg, x1, pre (1)	SR	SR	CR
Esen [49]	Methylprednisolone	IV	125 mg, x1, pre (1)	SR	SR	NR
Ustun [100]	Methylprednisolone	IV	1.5 mg/kg vs. 3 mg/kg, pre (1)	NCD	NCD	NCD

Abbreviations: CR, clinically responded; NCD, no clinical difference; NR, not reported; NSR, not statistically significant response; SR, statistically significant response.

prostaglandins. Examples include acetaminophen, aspirin, and cyclo-oxygenase (COX-1 and COX-2) nonsteroidal anti-inflammatory drugs (NSAIDs).

Perioperative opioid administration decreases pain, increases tolerance to pain, and provides a pleasant sedating effect. Opioids, however, are responsible for producing several adverse effects, such as respiratory depression, nausea, vomiting, constipation, allergic reaction, and increased tolerance. When comparing the analgesic efficacy of opioids, NSAIDs, and combinations of these medications, the combined formulations provided the highest efficacy. Opioids repeatedly have been shown to be less effective than NSAIDS in relieving pain after third molar removal [63–67] and are responsible for producing more adverse effects [63–68].

The mechanism of action of NSAIDs is to reduce production of peripheral prostaglandins,

thromboxane A2, and prostacycline production by inhibiting COX enzymes. Adverse effects of NSAIDs include bleeding, tinnitus, and renal failure. COX-1 receptors are found within all tissue, and COX-2 receptors are only present in inflammatory and neoplastic tissue [59,69]. The use of COX-2 inhibitors was initially favored over classical NSAIDs because of a 50% reduction in the side effects associated with NSAID administration, namely peptic ulcer disease and renal failure [47]. Unfortunately, it has been determined that COX-2 inhibitors induce thrombosis in patients with a history of coronary artery disease or cerebral vascular accidents. As a result, some of the COX-2 inhibitors have been withdrawn by the US Food and Drug Administration or the drug manufacturers.

In summary, the management of postoperative pain after third molar removal varies significantly.

Most surgeons administer perioperative intravenous (IV) corticosteroids to patients being sedated for the surgery. Many surgeons use a tapered oral steroid preparation in addition to or in lieu of perioperative dosing. All surgeons prescribe postoperative analgesics. The most common classes of medications are opioids and NSAIDs. The most common opioid preparations include oxycodone, hydrocodone, and acetaminophen and codeine. Ibuprofen is the most common NSAID prescribed. Nausea is the most frequently encountered adverse effect of opioids, and gastrointestinal pain and bleeding are the most common adverse effect of the NSAIDs. Taking the medications with small amounts of food often prevents these adverse effects. Patients should be encouraged to take analgesic medications at the onset of pain or discomfort rather than waiting until the pain becomes unbearable. Dependency is rare as the result of short-term use of opioids. Patients who have a history of or are suspected of being substance abusers should not be prescribed narcotics. NSAIDs can reduce third molar pain effectively in these patients, although the patients commonly insist that narcotics are required.

Nausea

Regardless of the type of surgical procedure performed, the primary perioperative concern for most patients was the development of nausea and vomiting. In fact, patients surveyed have indicated that they would rather deal with pain postoperatively than nausea and vomiting [70]. The overall prevalence of nausea and vomiting after general anesthesia has been estimated to be 25% to 30%, with 0.18% resulting in retractable nausea and vomiting [70]. The prevalence of nausea and vomiting after sedation procedures varies based on the depth and length of sedation. It has been determined that there is a lower risk for the development of nausea and vomiting from sedation than with general anesthesia [71]. In a prospective study conducted by Chye and colleagues [71], 1180 ambulatory surgery cases were performed with either general anesthesia or sedation and local anesthesia. Two thirds of the surgeries were performed with general anesthesia, and one third was performed with sedation. Postoperative nausea occurred in 14% of the cases performed with general anesthesia and in 6% of the cases performed with sedation and local anesthesia. In a much larger study presented by Perrott and colleagues [72], 71.9% of the cases were performed

by deep sedation or general anesthesia, 15.5% with conscious sedation, and 12.6% with local anesthesia. Third molar procedures represented 58.9% of the cases. The incidence of postoperative vomiting was 0.3%.

Vomiting is an objective finding defined as expulsion of gastrointestinal contents, whereas nausea is a subjective report provided by the patient and may not proceed to vomiting. The mechanisms responsible for vomiting involve activation of receptors in the lateral reticular formation of the medulla, which is in close proximity to the fourth ventricle, nucleus solitaries, and area postrema. These receptors may be activated by opiates, dopamine, enkephalin, serotonin, histamine, and acetylcholine. Nausea is typically prevented by various medications that act to block these receptors. The sequelae of postoperative nausea and vomiting include prolonged recovery time and patient dissatisfaction with the surgery. Physiologic adverse effects include elevated blood pressure with the risk of bleeding, aspiration, esophageal tear or rupture (Mallory Weis tear), and dehydration with electrolyte abnormalities, including hypokalemia, hypochloremia, hyponaturemia, and metabolic alkalosis. Known risk factors for the development of postoperative nausea and vomiting include age (beginning age 3 years, peak age 11–14, decreasing thereafter with increasing age), female gender (two to three times greater than for male patients), menstruation (increased risk within the first 7 days of menses), nonsmoking status, history of motion sickness (threefold increase), and previous history of postoperative nausea and vomiting [70,73,74].

Medications that induce nausea and vomiting include volatile anesthetics, nitrous oxide, and intravenous anesthetic agents, such as opiates [70]. Opiates cause an enhanced emetic effect by decreasing gastric motility and delaying gastric emptying. Intravenous anesthetic agents that provide rapid recovery, such as methohexital, have a higher incidence of nausea and vomiting than anesthetic agents such as thiopental, which provides a slower, smoother recovery. High-risk procedures for nausea and vomiting include strabismus repair, middle ear surgery, and gynecologic procedures [70]. Chemotherapy, radiation, hormonal imbalance (involving estrogen and progesterone), pregnancy, diabetes, elevated intracranial pressure, and uremia also increase the risk of nausea and vomiting [75,76]. The duration of sedation or anesthesia provided also affects the incidence of nausea and vomiting. Sinclair and

Table 3
Evaluation of analgesics and third molars

Study	Type	Groups	Result
Hepso [101]	Pre	1. Placebo 2. ASA 1000 mg	No decrease in postoperative pain, increased bleeding during and after surgery with ASA
Skelbred [102]	Pre and post	1. ASA 2. Acetaminophen	Increased bleeding with ASA, no difference in pain relief
Lokken [103]	Pre	1. Placebo 2. Ibuprofen	Decreased pain and swelling, no difference in bleeding
Dionne [64]	Pre and post	1. Ibuprofen pre vs. placebo 2. Ibuprofen post vs. ASA	Increased time needed for postoperative medication
Dionne [104]	Pre and post	1. Ibuprofen 800 mg pre and 400 mg post x2 2. Placebo and acetaminophen/codeine post 600/60	Ibuprofen group had significantly less pain
Hill [63]	Pre and post	1. Ibuprofen 2. Ibuprofen and codeine 3. Diflunisal	Ibuprofen decreased pain by 1.5–2 times
Amin [66]	Pre and post	1. Indomethacin 2. Codeine/acetaminophen 30/300 3. Placebo	Significant decrease with indomethacin 1/25 episode gastric upset
Dionne [105]	Pre and post	1. Flurbiprofen 50–100 2. Oxycodone 10/acetaminophen 650 mg	Flurbiprofen resulted in less adverse effect and greater analgesia
Dupuis [65]	Pre and post	1. Flurbiprofen 50 2. Codeine/ASA 3. Placebo	Greater analgesic effect with flurbiprofen preoperatively, equivocal postoperative effect
Hutchison [106]	Pre	1. Piroxicam 40 mg pre 2. Placebo	Significant less narcotic use in postoperative period
Graziani [107]	Pre	1. Piroxicam-FDDF 20 mg 2. Azithromycin 500 mg 3. 1 and 2	Proxicam with and without azithromycin provided better analgesia than azithromycin alone
Petersen [68]	Pre and post	1. Diflunisal 2. Codeine 3. Placebo	Diflunisal with superior analgesic efficacy in the first postoperative day, equivocal result on the third day
Bamgbose [108]	Pre	1. Dexamethasone 8 mg/4 mg 2. Diclofenac and dexamethasone	Group 2 with better pain relief and less facial swelling (up to 48 hr) $P > 0.05$, no change in trismus
Jung [109]	Pre and post PRN	Talniflumate 370 mg pre Talniflumate 370 mg post Talniflumate 370 mg PRN	Postoperative talniflumate provided better analgesia
Hersh [110]	Pre	1. Bromfenac 5 mg 2. Bromfenac 25 mg 3. Bromfenac 50 mg 4. Bromfenac 100 mg 5. Placebo	All except 5 mg produced statistically significant analgesic effects

(*continued on next page*)

Table 3 (*continued*)

Study	Type	Groups	Result
Van Dyke [111]	Post	1. Oxycodone 5 mg/ ibuprofen 400 mg 2. Oxycodone 5 mg 3. Ibuprofen 400 mg	Oxycodone 5 mg/ibuprofen 400 mg provided superior result; oxycodone alone was no more effective than placebo
Litkowski [67]	Post	1. Oxycodone 5 mg/ ibuprofen 400 mg 2. Oxycodone 5 mg/ acetaminophen 325 mg 3. Hydrocodone 7.5 mg/ acetaminophen 500 mg	Oxycodone 5 mg/ibuprofen 400 mg was superior treatment when compared to other treatment; $P < 0.001$
Ziccardi [112]	Post	1. Vicoprofen 2. Acetaminophen with codeine 3. Placebo	Vicoprofen was found to be superior to acetaminophen with codeine and placebo
Daniels [113]	Pre	1. Valdecoxib 10 2. Valdecoxib 20 3. Valdecoxib 40 4. Valdecoxib 80 5. Placebo	Longer duration of pain-free result, lower requirement of postoperative medications
Daniels [114]	Post	1. Valdecoxib 2. Oxycodone/APAP	Longer duration of analgesia with Valdecoxib
Daniels [114]	Post	1. Parecoxib 20 mg IM 2. Parecoxib 40 mg IM 3. Parecoxib 60 mg IM 4. Ketorolac 40 mg IV	Parecoxib provided analgesic efficacy comparable to ketorolac while providing duration of action
Moore [115]	Pre	1. Placebo 2. Rofecoxib 50 mg 3. Dexamethasone 10 mg 4. 2 and 3	Group 4 with reduced pain, trismus, and swelling compared to others; $P < 0.05$
Chiu [116]	Pre	1. Rofecoxib 50 mg 2. Ibuprofen 400 mg 3. Placebo	Rofecoxib provided better analgesics and longer duration for rescue medication compared to ibuprofen and placebo
Ong [117]	Pre vs. Post	1. Placebo before and rofecoxib after 2. Rofecoxib before and placebo after	Preoperative treatment with rofecoxib 50 mg provided superior analgesia when compared to postoperative treatment
Chang [118]	Pre	1. Rofecoxib 50 mg 2. Acetaminophen/codeine 600/60 mg	Rofecoxib was superior in pain reduction; $P < 0.001$
Ladov [119]	Post	1. Butorphanol nasal spray 4 mg and ibuprofen	Case series of butorphanol efficacious and well tolerated
Desjardins [120]	Post	1. Butorphanol nasal 0.25 mg 2. Butorphanol nasal 0.5 mg 3. Butorphanol nasal 1.0 mg 4. Butorphanol nasal 2 mg 5. Placebo	Significant analgesia with 1 and 2 mg intranasal route, two episodes of drowsiness and dizziness with 2.0 mg

Abbreviations: Pre, preoperative; Post, postoperative.

Mezei [77] indicated that for each 30-minute increase in the length of surgery, there is an increased risk of developing nausea and vomiting that amounts to 60% of the baseline. Increasing the time for surgery to more than 3 hours for a patient who is morbidly obese significantly increases the risk for postoperative nausea and vomiting [78].

Traditional antiemetics, such as scopolamine (anticholinergic), promethazine (phenothiazine), droperiodol (butyrophenones), diphenhydramine (antihistamine), and metoclopromide (benzamide), may produce numerous side effects, such as sedation, hypotension, extrapyramidal symptoms, dysphonic effects, and dry mouth. The newer medications, such as ondansetron, granistron, and dolasetron (serotonin receptor antagonists), have fewer adverse effects, such as headache and dizziness, but are far more expensive [79]. Nontraditional antiemetics consist of ephedrine, propofol, corticosteroids, and benzodiazepines. Except for ephedrine, the nontraditional antiemetics are commonly used in third molar surgery and subsequently reduce the prevalence of postoperative nausea and vomiting [70]. Prophylactic antiemetic therapy after sedation or general anesthesia for third molar surgery is a subject of controversy.

There is considerable variation in length and depth of anesthesia provided by oral and maxillofacial surgeons. The risk of postoperative nausea and vomiting after third molar surgery can vary. A simplified "risk scoring system" developed by Apfel and colleagues [80] may help to decide who would benefit from antiemetic prophylaxis. This system was based on a prospective study with 2722 adult patients (German and Danish) who underwent various procedures without antiemetics. Postoperative nausea and vomiting were assessed for 24 hours. The risk factors considered were female gender, nonsmoker status, motion sickness, prior postoperative nausea, and use of postoperative narcotics. When one, two, three, or four risk factors were present, the risk of postoperative nausea and vomiting was 10%, 21%, 39%, 61%, and 79%, respectively [80]. The patient may be given a score based on the number of risk factors assigned. This score may be beneficial in selecting prophylactic antiemetics before administration of sedation or general anesthesia for third molar surgery.

Nausea and vomiting after third molar removal is most commonly related to the sedation or the narcotic analgesics used for pain control. Promethazine, trimethobenzamide, and perchloroperazine given either orally or as a suppository are effective, inexpensive antiemetics. Ondansetron, a more effective antiemetic, comes in IV or oral form and is expensive.

Herbal supplements

The prevalence of herbal supplement consumption in the "third molar extraction population" is not known. Within the United States, 12.1% of the adult population currently uses herbal medication [81,82]. This number represents a significant increase when compared with 2.5% in 1990 [82]. In a recent survey of patients undergoing cosmetic surgery, twice as many patients reported using herbal supplements when compared with the general population [83]. In patients undergoing various inpatient or ambulatory procedures, the prevalence of herbal medication consumption was recorded as 22% and 32%, respectively [84,85]. The typical age for patients taking herbal supplementation is approximately 40, which represents a much older population than the typical patient undergoing third molar removal.

Perioperative use of herbal medication represents a significant concern because of the multiple pharmacologic and physiologic effects directed against the patient. Various effects, such as prolonged or inadequate anesthesia, inadequate anticoagulation, bleeding, stroke, or myocardial infarction, may be induced by medication interactions. Unfortunately, patients may not volunteer information regarding their use of herbal medication. Because most surgeons are poorly educated regarding alternative medicine, they are unaware of the side effects caused by herbal medications. In a recent study by Kaye and colleagues [84], 70% of patients failed to mention their use of herbal medicine. They believed that their physician would either have a poor knowledge of herbal medicine or be biased toward its benefits. The patients also believed that herbal medicine consumption would not affect the surgical outcome, which is a serious misconception by the public. Herbal medications are capable of causing serious adverse complications that may be either acute or chronic. Acute effects may be easier to identify. Adverse effects may present in certain populations because of concurrent medications, food, and specific genetic and racial backgrounds. Ultimately it is the responsibility of individual herbalists to inform patients of these side effects. These supplements are not regulated by the US FDA, which monitors each new

Table 4
Perioperative selected herbal medication adverse effects

Herbal medication	Indications	Adverse effects
Echinacea [86,121–123]	Treatment of infection, mostly upper respiratory tract, ulcer, arthritis, prevent bruising	Immunosuppression, decreases the effect of immunosupression medication, poor wound healing, allergic reaction
Ephedra (Ma Haung) [124–127] As of April 12, 2004 banned by FDA	Increased energy, appetite suppressant, bronchodilator	Insomnia, nausea, irritability, infarction, stop 24 hours before surgery
Garlic (active compound, allicin) [128,129]	Lower cholesterol, antibacterial and antimycotic, antithrombotic	Inhibits platelet aggression, prolongs bleeding, stop 7 days before surgery
Ginko [130–132]	Peripheral vascular disease, vertigo and tinnitus, cognitive disorder, erectile dysfunction	Increases bleeding, decreases blood clot formation, spontaneous hyphema, stop 36 hours before surgery
Ginseng [133,134]	Hemoptysis, gastric disturbance, stress, weakness, type II diabetes	Inhibits platelet aggression, increases risk of bleeding, hypoglycemia, discontinue 7 days before surgery
Kava [135,136]	Hypnosis, sedation, and analgesia, antispasmodic, anticonvulsant	Potentiates the effect of barbiturate and benzodiazepine, discontinue 24 hours before surgery
St. John Wort [137,138]	Anxiety, depression	Prolongs the effect of benzodiazepine, decreases cyclosporine level, increases the medication metabolism
Valerian [139]	Nervousness, depression, insomnia, GABA re-uptake inhibitor	Abrupt interruption may produce a withdrawal symptoms
Vitamin E [140]	Cardioprotective, antioxidant	Prolongs bleeding, inhibits wound healing
Saw palmetto [141]	Sedative, anti-inflammatory, benign prosthetic hypertrophy, aphrodisiac	Intraoperative bleeding, nausea, vomiting, diarrhea
Eicosapentaenoic acid (fish oil) [142]	Skin disorder, cardioprotective, asthma	ADPase inhibitor, prevents platelet aggregation
Condrotinin [83]	Osteoarthritis	Increases bleeding
Glucosamine [83]	Osteoarthritis	Hypoglycemia

medication for its adverse effects. The manufacturers are responsible for self-reporting adverse effects to the US FDA. Adverse effects of herbal medication may go unnoticed for a long period of time.

Some of the most commonly used herbal medicines are echinacea, ephedra, garlic, gingko, ginseng, kava, St. John's Wort, and valerian [86]. A summary of their common indications and adverse effects is contained in Table 4. These medications are considered "natural," organic, safe, and different than modern medicine prescribed by physicians. In modern medicine, however, more than 30% of prescribed medications are also obtained from plants [87]. Some examples include atropine (foxglove), vincristine (periwinkle), and salicylic acid (meadowsweet plant and white willow). Because of poor patient perception of herbal medicine and failure to share this information, it is the surgeon's responsibility to determine use of these substances during the preoperative interview.

Summary

Surgery is a stressful experience for many patients. Minimizing adverse side effects makes the surgical experience more favorable for patients. This article provides a literature review of various therapeutic agents used to minimize pain, edema, trismus, nausea, vomiting, infection, and adverse medication interactions. The risk factors for each adverse side effect are analyzed. Although the article does not advocate a particular guideline, it provides literature integrating various surgeons' findings. Dosing, route of administration, and comparative evaluation of various agents are

discussed. Each patient and each surgical procedure are different, however. Surgeons should assess
patient risk factors and surgical risk factors to
substantiate use of any chemotherapeutic agents.

References

[1] Cruse PJ, Foord R. The epidemiology of wound infection. Surg Clin North Am 1980;60:27–40.

[2] Woods RK, Dellinger EP. Current guidelines for
antibiotic prophylaxis of surgical wounds. Am
Fam Physician 1998;57(11):2731–40.

[3] Haley RW, Schaberg DR, Crossley KB, Von All-
men SD, et al. Extra charge and prolongation of
stay attributable to nosocomical infections: a prospective interhospital comparison. Am J Med
1981;70:51–8.

[4] Wenzel RP. Preoperative antibiotic prophylaxis.
N Engl J Med 1992;26:337–9.

[5] Dajani AS, Taubert KA, Wilson W, et al. Prevention of bacterial endocarditis: recommendations
by the American heart association. J Am Dent
Assoc 1997;128:1142–50.

[6] Deacon JM, Pagliaro AJ, Zelicof SB, et al. Prophylactic use of antibiotic for procedures after total
joint replacement. J Bone Joint Surg Am 1996;
78A:1755–71.

[7] Alexander JW. The contributions of infection control to a century of surgical progress. Ann Surg
1985;201:423.

[8] Burke JF. The effective period of preventive antibiotic action in experimental incisions and dermal
lesions. Surgery 1961;50:161–8.

[9] Classen DC, Evans RS, Pestotnik SL, et al. The
timing of prophylactic administration of antibiotics
and risk of surgical-wound infection. N Engl J Med
1992;326:281–6.

[10] Peterson LJ. Antibiotic prophylaxis against wound
infections in oral and maxillofacial surgery. J Oral
Maxillofac Surg 1990;48:617–20.

[11] White RP, Madianos PN, Offenbacher S, Blakey
GH, et al. Microbial complexes detected in the sec-
ond/third molar region in patients with asymptomatic third molars. J Oral Maxillofac Surg 2002;60:
1234–40.

[12] Calhoun NR. Dry socket and other postoperative
complications. Dent Clin North Am 1971;15:337.

[13] Osborn TP, Frederickson G, Small IA, Torgerson
TS. A prospective study of complications related
to mandibular third molar surgery. J Oral Maxillofac Surg 1985;43:767–9.

[14] Muhonen A, Venta I, Ylipaavalniemi P. Factors
predisposing to postoperative complications related to wisdom tooth surgery among university
students. J Am Coll Health 1971;46:39.

[15] Goldberg MH, Nemarich AN, Marco WP. Complications after mandibular third molar surgery:
a statistical analysis of 500 consecutive procedures

in private practices. J Am Dent Assoc 1985;111:
277.

[16] Haug RH, Perrott DH, Gonzalez ML, et al. The
American Association of Oral and Maxillofacial
Surgeons age-related third molar study. J Oral
Maxillofac Surg 2005;63:1106–14.

[17] Figueredo R, Valmaseda-Castellon E, Berini-Aytes
L, et al. Incidence and clinical features of delayed-
onset infections after extraction of lower third
molars. Oral Surg Oral Med Oral Pathol 2005;99:
265–9.

[18] Bui CH, Seldin EB, Dodson TB. Types, frequency
and risk factors for complications after third molar
extraction. J Oral Maxillofac Surg 2003;61:1379–89.

[19] Piecuch JF, Arzadon J, Lieblich SE. Prophylactic
antibiotics for third molar surgery: a supportive
opinion. J Oral Maxillofac Surg 1995;53:53–60.

[20] Chiapasco M, De Cicco L, Marrone G. Side effects and complications associated with third
molar surgery. Oral Surg Oral Med Oral Pathol
1993;76:412–20.

[21] Happonen RP, Backstorm AC, Ylipaavalniemi P.
Prophylactic use of phenoxymethylpenicillin and
tinidazole in mandibular third molar surgery:
a comparative placebo controlled clinical trial. Br
J Oral Maxillofac Surg 1990;28:12.

[22] Mitchell DA. A controlled clinical trial of prophylactic tinidazole for chemoprophylaxis in third
molar surgery. Br Dent J 1986;160:284.

[23] Mitchell DA, Morris TA. Tinidazole or pivampicil-
lin in third molar surgery. Int J Oral Maxillofac
Surg 1987;16:171–4.

[24] Sisk AL, Hammer WB, Shelton DW, et al. Complications following removal of impacted third molars. J Oral Maxillofac Surg 1986;44:855–9.

[25] Nordenram A, Sydnes G, Odegaard J. Neomycin-
baciteracin cones in impacted third molar sockets.
Int J Oral Maxillofac Surg 1973;2:279–83.

[26] Curran JB, Kennett S, Young AR. An assessment
of the use of prophylactic antibiotics in third molar
surgery. Int J Oral Surg 1974;3:1.

[27] Larsen PE. The effect of chlorhexidine rinse on the
incidence of alveolar osteitis following the surgical
removal of impacted mandibular third molars.
J Oral Maxillofac Surg 1991;49:932–7.

[28] Sweet JB, Butler DP. The relationship of smoking
to localized osteitis. J Oral Surg 1979;37:732–5.

[29] Meechan JG, Macgregor ID, Rogers SN, et al. The
effect of smoking on immediate post-extraction
socket filling with blood and the incidence of painful
socket. Br J Oral Maxillofac Surg 1988;26:402–9.

[30] Mitchell L. Topical metronidazole in the treatment
of "dry socket". Br Dent J 1984;156:132–4.

[31] Lyall JB. Third molar surgery: the effect of primary
closure, wound dressing and metroniadazole on
postoperative recovery. J R Army Med Corps
1991;137:100–3.

[32] Lloyd CJ, Earl PD. Metronidazole two or three
times daily: a comparative controlled clinical trial

of the efficacy of two different dosing schedules of metronidazole for chemoprophylaxis following third molar surgery. Br J Oral Maxillofac Surg 1994;32:165–7.

[33] Nitzan DNW. On the genesis of "dry socket". J Oral Maxillofac Surg 1983;13:15–22.

[34] Beirne OR, Hollander B. The effect of methylprednisolone on pain, trismus and swelling after removal of third molar. Oral Surg Oral Med Oral Pathol 1986;61:134.

[35] Laskin DM. Oral and maxillofacial surgery. St. Louis (MO): Mosby; 1985.

[36] Peterson LJ. Postoperative patient management. In: Peterson LJ, Ellis E, Hupp JR, Tucker MR, editors. Contemporary oral and maxillofacial surgery. 3rd edition. St Louis (MO): Mosby; 1998: 251.

[37] Messer EJ, Keller JJ. The use of intraoral dexamethasone after extraction of mandibular third molars. Oral Surg Oral Med Oral Pathol 1975;40: 594–8.

[38] Hench PS, Kendall EC, Slocumb CH, et al. The effect of a hormone of the adrenal cortex (17-hydroxy-11dehdrocorticosterone; compound E) and of pituitary adrenocorticotropic hormone on rheumatoid arthritis. Proceedings of the Staff Meeting of the Mayo Clinic 1949;24:181.

[39] Melby JC. Adrenocorticosteroids in medical emergencies. Med Clin North Am 1961;45:875.

[40] Gersema L, Baker K. Use of corticosteroids in oral surgery. J Oral Maxillofac Surg 1992;48:179–87.

[41] Little JW, Falace D, Miller C, et al. Adrenal insufficiency. In: Dental management of the medically compromised patient. St Louis (MO): Mosby; 1988.

[42] Melby JC. Clinical pharmacology of systemic corticosteroids. Annu Rev Pharmacol Toxicol 1977;17: 511–27.

[43] Montgomery MH, Hogg JP, Roberts DL, et al. The use of glucocorticosteroids to lessen the inflammatory sequelae following third molar surgery. J Oral Maxillofac Surg 1990;48:179–87.

[44] Koerner KR. Steroid in third molar surgery: a review. Gen Dent 1987;35:459–63.

[45] Bahn SL. Glucocorticosteroids in dentistry. J Am Dent Assoc 1982;105:476–81.

[46] Axelrod L. Glucocorticoid therapy. Medicine 1979; 55:39.

[47] Fitzgerald GA, Patrono C. Drug therapy: the coxibs, selective inhibitors of cyclooxygenase-2. N Engl J Med 2001;345:433–42.

[48] Milles M, Desjardins PJ. Reduction of postoperative facial swelling by low-dose methylprednisolone. J Oral Maxillofac Surg 1993;51:987–91.

[49] Esen E, Tasar F, Akhan O. Determination of the anti-inflammatory effects of methylprednisolone on sequelae of third molar surgery. J Oral Maxillofac Surg 1999;57:1201–6.

[50] Sisk AL, Bonnington GJ. Evaluation of methylprednisolone and flurbiprofen for inhibition for

the postoperative inflammatory response. Oral Surg Oral Med Oral Pathol 1985;60:137.

[51] Huffman G. Use of methylprednisolone sodium succinate to reduce postoperative edema after removal of impacted third molars. J Oral Surg 1977;35:1977.

[52] Axelrod L. Adrenal corticosteroids. In: Miller RR, Greenblatt DJ, editors. Handbook for drug therapy. New York: Elsevier; 1979.

[53] Ross R, White CP. Evaluation of hydrocortisone in prevention of postoperative complications after oral surgery: a preliminary report. J Oral Surg 1958;16:220.

[54] Hooley JR, Hohl T. Use of steroids in the prevention of some complications after traumatic oral surgery. J Oral Surg 1974;32:864.

[55] Alexander RE, Throndson RR. A review of perioperative corticosteroid use in dentoalveolar surgery. Oral Surg Oral Med Oral Pathol 2000;90: 406–15.

[56] Claman HN. Glucocorticosteroids II: the clinical responses. Hosp Pract 1982;18:143.

[57] Byyny RL. Withdraw from glucocorticoid therapy. N Engl J Med 1976;295:30.

[58] Leshin M. Acute adrenal insufficiency: recognition, management and prevention. Urol Clin North Am 1982;9:229.

[59] Savage MG, Henry MA. Preoperative nonsteroidal anti-inflammatory agents: review of the literature. Oral Surg Oral Med Oral Pathol Oral Radiol Endod 2004;98:146–52.

[60] Hardy JD, Wolfe HG, Goodell H. Experimental evidence on the nature of cutaneous hyperalgesia. J Clin Invest 1950;29:115–40.

[61] Treede RD, Meyer RA, Raja SN, Campbell JN, et al. Peripheral and central mechanism of cutaneous hyperalgesia. Prog Neurobiol 1992;38:397–421.

[62] Dray A. Kinins and their receptors in hyperalgesia. Can J Physiol Pharmacol 75:704–12.

[63] Hill CM, Carroll MJ, Giles AD, et al. Ibuprofen given pre- and post-operatively for the relief of pain. Int J Oral Maxillofac Surg 1987;16:420–4.

[64] Dionne RA, Cooper SA. Evaluation of preoperative ibuprofen for postoperative pain after removal of third molars. Oral Surg Oral Med Oral Pathol Oral Radiol Endod 1978;1978:851–6.

[65] Dupuis R, Lemay H, Bushnetter MC, et al. Preoperative flurbiprofen in oral surgery: a method of choice in controlling postoperative pain. Pharmacotherapy 1988;8:193–200.

[66] Amin MM, Laskin DM. Prophylactic use of indomethacin for prevention of post surgical complications after removal of impacted third molars. Oral Surg Oral Med Oral Pathol Oral Radiol Endod 1983;55:448–51.

[67] Litkowski LJ, Christensen SE, Adamson DN, et al. Analgesic efficacy and tolerability of oxycodone 5mg/ibuprofen 400 mg compared with those of oxycodone 5 mg/acetaminophen 325 mg and

hydrocodone 7.5 mg/acetaminophen 500 mg in patients with moderate to severe postoperative pain: a randomized, double-blind placebo-controlled, single-dose parallel-group study in a dental pain model. Clin Ther 2005;27:418–29.

[68] Petersen JK. The analgesic and anti-inflammatory efficacy of diflunisal and codeine after removal of impacted third molars. Curr Med Res Opin 1978; 5:525–35.

[69] Vane JR, Bakhle YS, Botting RM. Cyclooxygenase 1 and 2. Annu Rev Pharmacol Toxicol 1998;38: 97–120.

[70] Kovac AL. Prevention and treatment of postoperative nausea and vomiting. Drugs 2000;59(2): 213–43.

[71] Chye EP, Young IG, Osborne GA, et al. Outcomes after same-day surgery: a review of 1180 cases at a major teaching hospital. J Oral Maxillofac Surg 1993;51(8):846–9.

[72] Perrot DH, Yuen JP, Andresen RV, et al. Office-based ambulatory anesthesia: outcomes of clinical practices of oral and maxillofacial surgeons. J Oral Maxillofac Surg 2003;61(9):983–95.

[73] Kovac AL. The prophylactic treatment of postoperative nausea and vomiting in oral and maxillofacial surgery. J Oral Maxillofac Surg 2005;63:1531–5.

[74] Honkavarra P, Lehtinen AM, Hovorka J, et al. Nausea and vomiting after gynecological laparoscopy depends upon the phase of the menstrual cycle. Can J Anaesth 1991;38:876–9.

[75] Haigh CG, Kaplan LA, Durham JM, et al. Nausea and vomiting after gynecological surgery: a meta-analysis of factors affecting their incidence. Br J Anaesth 1993;71:512–22.

[76] Philip BK. Etiologies of postoperative nausea and vomiting. Pharmacy Ther 1997;22:512–22.

[77] Sinclair DR, Chung F, Mezei G. Can postoperative nausea and vomiting be predicted? Anesthesiology 1999;91:109.

[78] Watcha MF, White FP. Postoperative nausea and vomiting: its etiology, treatment and prevention. Anesthesiology 1992;1992:162–84.

[79] McNiece WL. Practical solutions for difficult problems: II. Drug cost analysis data in anesthesia. Anesthesiol Clin North Am 1996;14:573.

[80] Apfel CC, Laara E, Koivuranta M, et al. A simplified risk score for predicating postanesthetic nausea and vomiting. Anesthesiology 1999;91: 693–700.

[81] De Smet PA. Herbal remedies. N Engl J Med 2002; 347(5):2046–56.

[82] Eisenberg DM, Davis RB, Ettner SL, et al. Trends in alternative medicine use in the United States, 1990–1997: results of a follow-up national survey. JAMA 1998;280:1569–75.

[83] Heller J, Gabbay JS, Ghadjar K, et al. Top-10 list of herbal and supplemental medicines used by cosmetic patients: what the plastic surgeon needs to know. Plast Reconstr Surg 2006;117(2):436–45.

[84] Kaye AD, Clarke RC, Sabar R, et al. Herbal medication: current trends in anesthesiology practice a hospital survey. J Clin Anesth 2000; 12:468–71.

[85] Tsen LC, Segal S, Pothier M, et al. Alternative medicine use in presurgical patients. Anesthesiology 2000;93:148–51.

[86] Melchart D, Linde K, Fischer P, et al. Echinacea for prevention and treating the common cold. Cochran Database Syst Rev 2000;2:CD000530.

[87] Kleiner SM. The true nature of herbs. Sports Med 1995;23:13.

[88] Ware WH, Campvell JC, Taylor RC. Effect of a steroid on post operative swelling and trismus. Dent Prog 1963;3:116.

[89] Mead SV, Lynch DF, Mead SG. Triamcinolone given orally to control postoperative reactions to oral surgery. J Oral Surg 1964;22:484.

[90] Linenberg WB. The clinical evaluation of dexamethasone in oral surgery. Oral Surg Oral Med Oral Pathol 1965;20:6.

[91] Nathanson NR, Seifert DM. Betamethasone in dentistry. Oral Surg Oral Med Oral Pathol 1964; 18:715.

[92] Caci F, Gluck GM. Double-blind study of prednisolone and papase as inhibitors of complications after oral surgery. J Am Dent Assoc 1976;93:325.

[93] Bystedt H, Nordenram A. Effect of methylprednisolone on complications after removal of impacted mandibular third molars. Swed Dent J 1985;9(2): 65–9.

[94] Messer EJ, Keller JJ. The use of dexamethasone after extraction of mandibular third molars. Oral Surg 1975;40:594.

[95] Edilby GI, Canniff JP, Harris M. Double-blind placebo-controlled trial of the effects of dexamethasone on postoperative swelling. J Dent Res 1982; 61:556.

[96] Skejelbred P, Lokken P. Postoperative pain and inflammatory reaction reduced by injection of a corticosteroid. Eur J Clin Pharmacol 1982;21:391.

[97] Skejelbred P, Lokken P. Reduction of pain and swelling by corticosteroid injected three hours after surgery. Eur J Clin Pharmacol 1985;23:141.

[98] El Hag M, Coghlan K, Christmas P, et al. The anti-inflammatory effects of dexamethasone and therapeutic ultrasound in oral surgery. Br J Oral Maxillofac Surg 1985;23:17.

[99] Pederson A. Decadronphosphate in the relief of complaint after third molar surgery. Int J Oral Maxillofac Surg 1985;14:235.

[100] Ustun Y, Erdogan O, Esen E, et al. Comparison of the effects of 2 doses of methylprednisolone on pain, swelling and trismus after third molar surgery. Oral Surg Oral Med Oral Pathol Oral Radiol Endod 2003;96:535–9.

[101] Hepso HU, Lokken P, Bjornson J, et al. Double blind crossover study of the effect of acetylsalicylic acid on bleeding and postoperative course after

bilateral oral surgery. Eur J Clin Pharmacol 1976; 10:217–25.

[102] Skjelbred P, Album B, Lokken P. Acetylsalicylic acid vs. paracetamol effects on post-operative course. Eur J Clin Pharmacol 1976;12:257–69.

[103] Loken P, Olsen I, Bruaset I, et al. Bilateral surgical removal of impacted lower third molar teeth as a model for drug evaluation: a test with ibuprofen. Eur J Clin Pharmacol 1975;8:209–16.

[104] Dionne RA, Campbell RA, Cooper SA, et al. Suppression of postoperative pain by preoperative administration of ibuprofen in comparison to placebo, acetaminophen and acetaminophen plus codeine. J Clin Pharmacol 1983;23:37–43.

[105] Dionne RA, Sisk AL, Fox PC. Suppression of postoperative pain by preoperative administration of flurbiprofen in comparison to acetaminophen and oxycodone plus acetaminophen. Curr Med Res 1983;34:15–29.

[106] Hutchison GL, Crofts SL, Gray IG. Preoperative piroxicam for postoperative analgesia in dental surgery 1990;65:500–3.

[107] Graziani F, Corsi L, Fornai M, et al. Clinical evaluation of piroxicam-FDDF and azithromycin in the prevention of complications associated with impacted lower third molar extraction. Pharmacol Res 2005;52:485–90.

[108] Bamgbose BO, Akinwande JA, Adeyemo WL, et al. Effects of co-administrated dexamethasone and diclofenac potassium on pain, swelling and trismus following third molar surgery. Head Face Med 2005;1:11.

[109] Jung YS, Kim MK, Um YJ, et al. The effects on postoperative oral surgery pain by varying NSAIDS administration times: comparison on effect of preemptive analgesia. Oral Surg Oral Med Oral Pathol Oral Radiol Endod 2005;100:559–63.

[110] Hersh EV, Cooper SA, Levin LM, et al. A dose-ranging study of bromfenac sodium in oral surgery pain. Oral Surg Oral Med Oral Pathol Oral Radiol Endod 1998;86:36–41.

[111] Van Dyke T, Litkowski LJ, Kiersch TA, et al. Combination oxycodone 5mg/ibuprofen 400 mg for the treatment of postoperative pain: a double-blind, placebo-and active-controlled parallel-group study. Clin Ther 2004;26(12):2003–14.

[112] Ziccardi VB, Desjardins PJ, Daly-DeJoy E, et al. Single-dose vicoprofen compared with acetaminophen with codeine and placebo in patients with acute postoperative pain after third molar extractions. J Oral Maxillofac Surg 2000;58:622–8.

[113] Daniels SE, Talwalker S, Hubbard RC, et al. Preoperative valdecoxib, a COX-2 specific inhibitor, provides effective and long lasting pain relief following oral surgery. Presented at the Annual Meeting of the American Society of Anesthesiologists. New Orleans, LA; October 2001.

[114] Daniels SE, Desjardins PJ, Talwalker S, et al. The analgesic efficacy of valdecoxib vs. oxycodone/acetaminophen after oral surgery. J Am Dent Assoc 2002;133:611–21.

[115] Moore PA, Brar P, Smiga ER, et al. Preemptive rofecoxib and dexamethasone for prevention of pain and trismus following third molar surgery. Oral Surg Oral Med Oral Pathol Oral Radiol Endod 2005;99:E1–7.

[116] Chiu WK, Cheung LK. Efficacy of preoperative oral rofecoxib in pain control for third molar surgery. Oral Surg Oral Med Oral Pathol Oral Radiol Endod 2005;99:E47–53.

[117] Ong KS, Seymour RA, Yeo JF, et al. The efficacy of preoperative versus postoperative rofecoxib for preventing acute postoperative dental pain: a prospective randomized crossover study using bilateral symmetrical oral surgery. Clin J Pain 2005;21(6): 536–42.

[118] Chang DJ, Bird SR, Bohidar NR, et al. Analgesic efficacy of rofecoxib compared with codeine/acetaminophen using a model of acute dental pain. Oral Surg Oral Med Oral Pathol Oral Radiol Endod 2005;2005:E74–80.

[119] Ladov MJ, Precheur HV, Rauch DM, et al. An open-label evaluation of the efficacy and safety of stadol NS with ibuprofen in the treatment of pain after removal of impacted wisdom teeth. J Oral Maxillofac Surg 2000;58:15–8.

[120] Desjardins PJ, Norris LH, Cooper SA, et al. Analgesic efficacy of intranasal butorphanol in the treatment of pain after dental impaction surgery. J Oral Maxillofac Surg 2000;58:19–26.

[121] Gruenwald J, Brendler T, Jaenicke C. Echinacea. In: PDR for Herbal Medicines. 2000. p. 261–6.

[122] Peppin J. Echinacea. Am J Health Syst Pharm 1999;56:121–2.

[123] Braunin B. Echinacea purpurea radix for strengthening the immune response in flu-like infections. Z Phytother 1992;13:7.

[124] Nightingale SL. From the Food and Drug Administration. JAMA 1997;278:15.

[125] Haller CA, Benowitz NL. Adverse cardiovascular and central nervous system events associated with dietary supplements containing ephedra alkaloids. N Engl J Med 2000;343:1833–8.

[126] Ang-Lee MK, Moss J, Yuan CS. Herbal medicine and perioperative care. JAMA 2001;285:208–16.

[127] Zahn KA, Li RL, Purssell RA. Cardiovascular toxicity after ingestion of herbal ecstasy. J Emerg Med 1999;17(2):289–91.

[128] Srivastava KC. Evidence for the mechanism by which garlic inhibits platelet aggression. Prostaglandins Leukot Med 1986;22:313–21.

[129] Ali M, Al-Qattan KK, Al-Enezi F, et al. Khanafer RM, et al. Effect of allicin from garlic powder on serum lipids and blood pressure in rats fed with a high cholesterol diet. Prostaglandins Leukot Essent Fatty Acids 2000;62:463–8.

[130] Le Bars PL, Katz MM, Berman N, et al. A placebo-controlled double-blind randomized trial of

an extract of Ginkgo biloba for dementia: North American EGB Study Group. JAMA 1997;278: 1327–32.

[131] Fessenden JM, Wittenborn W, Clarke L. Gingko biloba: a case report of herbal medicine and bleeding post operatively from a laparoscopic cholecystectomy. Am Surg 2001;67:33–5.

[132] Rosenblatt M, Mindel J. Spontaneous hyphema associated with ingestion of gingko biloba extract. N Engl J Med 1997;336:1108.

[133] Kuo SC, Teng CM, Lee JC, et al. Antiplatelet components in panax ginseng. Planta Med 1990;56: 164–7.

[134] Attele AS, Wu JA, Yuan CS. Ginseng pharmacology: multiple constituents and multiple actions. Biochem Pharmacol 1999;58:1685–93.

[135] Peppin J. Kava: piper methysticum. Am J Health Syst Pharm 1999;56:957–8.

[136] Pittler MH, Ernst E. Efficacy of kava extract for treating anxiety: systemic review and meta-analysis. J Clin Psychopharmacol 2000;20:84–9.

[137] Gaster B, Holroyd J. St. John's Wort for depression: a systemic review. Arch Intern Med 2000;160:152–6.

[138] Shelton RC, Keller MB, Gelenberg A, et al. Effectiveness of St. John's Wort in major depression. JAMA 2001;2001:1978–86.

[139] Houghton PJ. The scientific basis for the reputed activity of valerian. J Pharm Pharmacol 1999;51:505–12.

[140] Havlik R. Vitamin E and wound healing: plastic surgery. Educational Foundation DATA Committee. Plast Reconstr Surg 1997;100:1901.

[141] Cheema P, El-Mefty O, Jazieh AR. Intraoperative hemorrhage associated with the use of extract of saw palmetto herb: a case report and review of literature. J Intern Med 2001;250:167.

[142] Awang DVC. Ginger. Can Pharm J 1992;309–11.

ELSEVIER
SAUNDERS

Oral Maxillofacial Surg Clin N Am 19 (2007) 85–91

ORAL AND
MAXILLOFACIAL
SURGERY CLINICS
of North America

Partial Odontectomy

M. Anthony Pogrel, DDS, MD, FRCS, FACS

*Department of Oral and Maxillofacial Surgery, University of California, San Francisco,
Box 0440, Room C-522, 521 Parnassus Avenue, San Francisco,
CA 94143-0440, USA*

The problem of inferior alveolar nerve involvement during the removal of lower third molars is a clinical and, more recently, medicolegal issue. Because the results of damage to the inferior alveolar nerve are unpredictable in that many cases do recover but some do not, it is preferable to carry out a technique that may reduce the possibility of this involvement. The technique of coronectomy, partial odontectomy, or deliberate root retention, is one such technique to protect the inferior alveolar nerve that has been studied intermittently in the past [1–8] but currently does not enjoy a strong body of support. In theory, retention of the apical portion of the roots of the lower third molar might be appropriate if preoperative imaging indicates an intimate relationship between the root of the tooth and the inferior alveolar nerve. Previously, the relationship between the roots of the mandibular teeth and inferior alveolar nerve were assessed radiographically, particularly with a panoramic radiograph. Studies have shown that on a panorex radiograph diversion of the inferior alveolar canal, darkening of the root interruption of the white line of the canal, narrowing of the canal, and deflection of the roots indicated a possible intimate nerve relationship to the tooth [9–11]. In the prospective study by Rood and Shehab [11] of 125 teeth with signs suggesting an increased risk of nerve involvement, 14% developed a nerve injury. Currently, however, with the advent of low-dose cone beam CT technology, which is becoming generally available throughout the United States in a dental outpatient setting, accurate three-dimensional imaging can be performed to show in detail the relationship between the inferior alveolar nerve and the lower third molars (Fig. 1) [12–15]. In this way, an objective decision can be made of cases in which there truly is contact between the nerve and the tooth and in which the technique of coronectomy might be advantageous.

Currently, and in the current state of knowledge, when a panorex radiograph suggests a relationship between the inferior alveolar nerve and the roots of the lower third molar, cone beam CT scanning should be advised for cases in which the results might influence the treatment to be performed. In cases in which an intimate relationship is confirmed, the technique of coronectomy merits consideration.

The intention of coronectomy or deliberate root retention is that the part of the root intimately related to the inferior alveolar nerve is undisturbed. Enough of the root must be removed below the crest of the lingual and buccal plates of bone to enable bone to form over the retained roots as part of the normal healing process, however. It is also believed to be important not to mobilize the roots, because they might damage the nerve and then become mobile foreign bodies.

Contraindications to coronectomy

The following factors are contraindications to coronectomy:

When the teeth have active infection around them, particularly infection involving the radicular portion of the tooth.

Teeth that are mobile should be excluded from this technique, because any retained roots may act as a mobile foreign body and become a nidus for infection or migration.

E-mail address: tony.pogrel@ucsf.edu

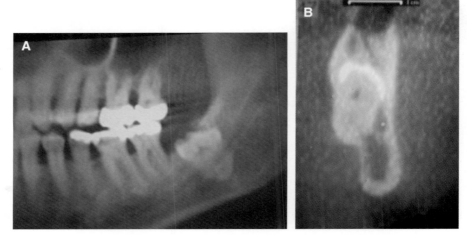

Fig. 1. A Panorex radiograph (*A*) and a cone beam CT scan (*B*) shows the relationship of the inferior alveolar nerve to the roots of a third molar in three dimensions. With both images, treatment can be customized appropriately. Note the virtual absence of the lingual plate and the lingual inclination of the tooth on the coronal CT scan.

Teeth that are horizontally impacted along the course of the inferior alveolar nerve may be unsuitable for this technique, because sectioning of the tooth itself could endanger the nerve (Fig. 2). The technique is better used with vertical, mesioangular, or distoangular impactions, in which the sectioning itself does not endanger the nerve.

Technique

All patients are placed on appropriate preoperative prophylactic antibiotics so that

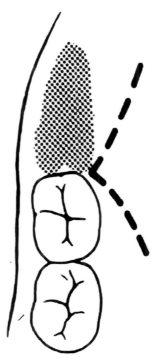

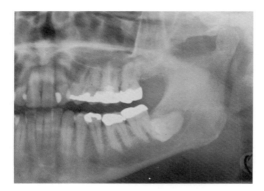

Fig. 2. A third molar lying horizontally along the inferior alveolar nerve. It would be difficult in this case to remove part of the tooth without endangering the inferior alveolar nerve.

Fig. 3. A conventional buccal incision left side along the external oblique ridge to the distobuccal line angle of the second molar and a releasing incision into the sulcus.

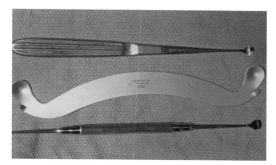

Fig. 4. A Walters-type lingual retractor with appropriate periosteal elevators to retract the lingual flap.

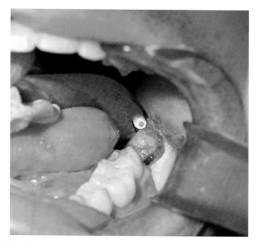

Fig. 6. A case in which complete sectioning of the tooth with a fissure bur led to grooving and even perforation of the lingual plate. This reinforces the importance of using a lingual retractor. (*From* Pogrel MA, Lee JS, Muff DF. Coronectomy: a technique to protect the inferior alveolar nerve. J Oral Maxillofac Surg 2004;62(12):1447–52; with permission. © Copyright 2004 – The American Association of Oral and Maxillofacial Surgeons.)

antibiotics are in the pulp chamber of the tooth to be sectioned. A conventional buccal incision with the raising of a buccal flap with releasing incision is used. The flap is elevated and retained with a Minnesota-type retractor (Fig. 3). A lingual flap is raised without tension on the lingual nerve, and the lingual tissues are retracted with an appropriate lingual retractor. A Walters-type lingual retractor is appropriate (Fig. 4).

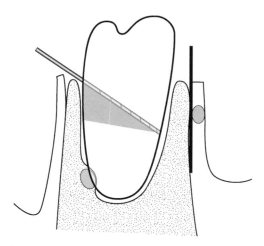

Fig. 5. Diagrammatic representation of coronectomy technique. A lingual retractor is in place to protect the lingual soft tissues, including the lingual nerve, and the fissure bur is used at approximately 45° to section the crown completely. The gray area is then removed secondarily to place the apical portion of the tooth at least 2 to 3 mm below the crest of bone. (*From* Pogrel MA, Lee JS, Muff DF. Coronectomy: a technique to protect the inferior alveolar nerve. J Oral Maxillofac Surg 2004;62(12):1447–52; with permission. © Copyright 2004 - The American Association of Oral and Maxillofacial Surgeons.)

Using a 701-type fissure bur, the crown of the tooth is transected at an angle of approximately 45° (Fig. 5). The crown is totally transected so that it can be removed with tissue forceps alone and does not need to be fractured from the roots. This approach minimizes the possibility of mobilizing the roots. For this technique to be effective, a lingual retractor is essential because the lingual plate of bone can be inadvertently perforated, and otherwise the lingual nerve would be at risk (Fig. 6). The Walters retractor (KLS Martin, Jacksonville, Florida) is a suitable instrument because it has no sharp edges, is shaped to fit the lingual aspect of the mandible, and has an extension that engages the internal oblique ridge and prevents the retractor from passing too far inferiorly (Fig. 7) [16].

After removal of the crown of the tooth, the fissure bur is used to reduce the remaining root fragments so that the remaining roots are at least 3 mm below the crest of the lingual and buccal plates in all dimensions. This involves removing the shaded portion in Fig. 5 (Fig. 8). There is no attempt at root canal treatment or any other therapy to the exposed vital pulp of the tooth.

A periosteal release must be performed so that a buccal flap can be advanced to obtain a watertight primary closure of the socket using one or more vertical mattress sutures. For accurate

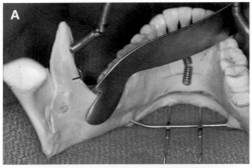

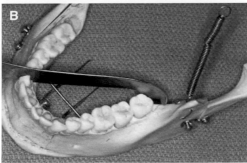

Fig. 7. (*A* and *B*) Models show lingual retractor in place to demonstrate that the shape of the lingual retractor fits the lingual contours of the mandible. The lip engages the internal oblique ridge and prevents the retractor from passing too far inferiorly.

record-keeping purposes, a radiograph should be taken postoperatively to show the size and position of the retained fragment.

Alternative techniques

For surgeons who do not wish—for various reasons—to place a lingual retractor, the following alternative techniques have been suggested. To raise a buccal flap only, section the crown two thirds of the way across toward the lingual side as in any normal third molar removal and then fracture off the crown of the tooth. Unfortunately, this technique can lead to mobilization and loosening of the root fragment, and in one study up to 30% of root fragments were mobilized by this technique and required removal at the same time as the crown [7]. It is possible on occasion to carry out the technique raising a buccal flap only and removing the crown of the tooth with a round bur in a high-speed handpiece from the occlusal aspect until enough of the tooth has been removed, but it is 3 mm below the buccal and

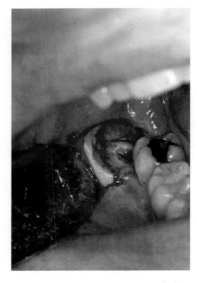

Fig. 8. The postoperative appearance of the coronectomy procedure shows the retained apical portion of the tooth 3 mm or more beneath the crest of bone. (*From* Pogrel MA, Lee JS, Muff DF. Coronectomy: a technique to protect the inferior alveolar nerve. J Oral Maxillofac Surg 2004;62(12):1447–52; with permission. © Copyright 2004 – The American Association of Oral and Maxillofacial Surgeons.)

lingual crest of bone. This technique, however, tends to take longer than sectioning with a fissure bur and leaves more tooth debris to be removed.

Results

Relatively few large or long-term studies of this technique have been performed, and reports of the literature are fairly brief. In our own institution, however, we have performed more than 300 of these cases. Our longest follow-up in this study is 7.5 years, and the mean follow-up is 5 years. To date, follow-up radiographs (taken at 6 months, 1 year, and 2 years postoperatively) have shown that in approximately 30% of cases there is genuine coronal migration of the root fragments away from the inferior alveolar nerve (Fig. 9). It can be surmised in these cases that the nerve does not actually perforate the root, otherwise it is assumed that coronal migration could not occur. In only one patient to date have these coronally migrating root apices needed to be removed. In only one case was there a failure to heal primarily after surgery, and in that case the root fragments on both sides were later removed and found to be mobile. The

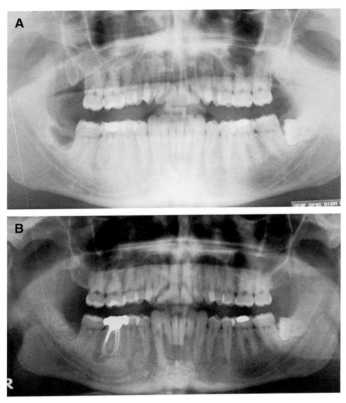

Fig. 9. (*A*) Immediate postcoronectomy radiograph shows retained apical portion of the lower right third molar. (*B*) Appearance 6 months later shows that the roots of the lower right third molar have migrated toward the occlusal plane and are no longer in apparent contact with the inferior alveolar nerve. (From: Pogrel MA, Lee JS, Muff DF. Coronectomy: a technique to protect the inferior alveolar nerve. J Oral Maxillofac Surg 2004;62(12):1447–52; with permission. © Copyright 2004 – The American Association of Oral and Maxillofacial Surgeons.)

6-month radiographs tend to show that the bone does form over the retained roots in most cases, although this occurrence has not been confirmed clinically in any cases (Fig. 10). It is assumed that the roots remain vital and no cases have required any root canal therapy.

Discussion

The technique of coronectomy seems to be a safe and straightforward technique with few complications or potential complications. In our own patients, there has only been one case of mild, transient (5 days) lingual paresthesia, presumably caused by the lingual retraction, but no other cases of lingual nerve involvement were reported. Other studies, however, have suggested a higher rate of transient lingual paresthesias from the use of the lingual retractor but not permanent cases of lingual nerve involvement [17–19]. There

does not seem to be any need to treat the exposed pulp of the tooth, and root treatment actually seems to be contraindicated. Animal studies have shown that vital roots remain vital with minimal degenerative changes [20–23]. Osteocementum usually extends to cover the roots.

The technique of leaving the retained root fragments at least 3 mm inferior to the crest of bone seems appropriate and seems to encourage bone formation over the retained root fragments. The distance of 2 to 3 mm has been validated in animal studies [21–23].

Late migration of the root fragments seems to occur in some cases, but it is unpredictable, and even if it does occur, the roots move further away from the nerve and into a safer position and are more easily removed later, if required. It seems that the final rates of root removal may be remarkably low, particularly when bone has grown over the roots.

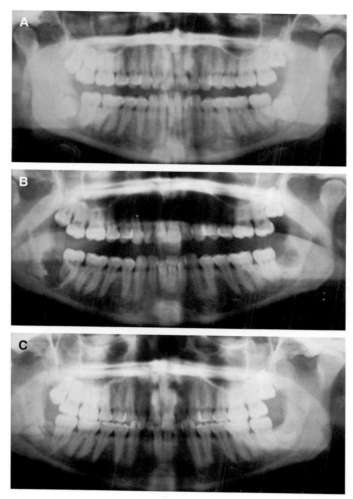

Fig. 10. (*A*) Appearance of tooth number 32 preoperatively shows an apparently intimate relationship with the inferior alveolar nerve and a dentigerous cyst present on the crown of the tooth. (*B*) Appearance immediately after coronectomy and simultaneous cystectomy. (*A* and *B From* Pogrel MA, Lee JS, Muff DF. Coronectomy: a technique to protect the inferior alveolar nerve. J Oral Maxillofac Surg 2004;62(12):1447–52; with permission. © Copyright 2004 – The American Association of Oral and Maxillofacial Surgeons.) (*C*) Appearance 1 year later shows the apical portion of the roots still in position, with bone having formed in the previous cystic cavity and coronal to the root fragments. This appearance demonstrates that this technique is applicable even in the presence of some types of pathology.

In summary, the technique of coronectomy is worthy of consideration in cases in which panorex radiograph and cone beam CT scanning show an intimate relationship between the roots of the mandibular third molar and the inferior alveolar nerve.

References

[1] Alantar A, Roisin-Chausson MH, Commissionat Y, et al. Retention of third molar roots to prevent damage to the inferior alveolar nerve. Oral Surg Oral Med Oral Pathol Oral Radiol Endod 1995; 80(2):126.

[2] Freedman GL. Intentional partial odontectomy: report of case. J Oral Maxillofac Surg 1992;50(4): 419–21.

[3] Freedman GL. Intentional partial odontectomy: review of cases. J Oral Maxillofac Surg 1997;55(5): 524–6.

[4] Knutsson K, Lysell L, Rohlin M. Postoperative status after partial removal of the mandibular third molar. Swed Dent J 1989;13(1–2):15–22.

[5] O'Riordan BC. Coronectomy (intentional partial odontectomy of lower third molars). Oral Surg Oral Med Oral Pathol Oral Radiol Endod 2004; 98(3):274–80.

[6] Pogrel MA, Lee JS, Muff DF. Coronectomy: a technique to protect the inferior alveolar nerve. J Oral Maxillofac Surg 2004;62(12):1447–52.

[7] Renton T, Hankins M, Sproate C, et al. A randomised controlled clinical trial to compare the incidence of injury to the inferior alveolar nerve as a result of coronectomy and removal of mandibular third molars. Br J Oral Maxillofac Surg 2005;43(1):7–12.

[8] Zola MB. Avoiding anesthesia by root retention. J Oral Maxillofac Surg 1993;51(8):954.

[9] Blaeser BF, August MA, Donoff RB, et al. Panoramic radiographic risk factors for inferior alveolar nerve injury after third molar extraction. J Oral Maxillofac Surg 2003;61(4):417–21.

[10] Howe G, Poynton HG. Prevention of damage to the inferior alveolar nerve during the evaluation of mandibular third molars. Br Dent J 1960;109:355–63.

[11] Rood JP, Shehab BA. The radiological prediction of inferior alveolar nerve injury during third molar surgery. Br J Oral Maxillofac Surg 1990;28(1):20–5.

[12] Danforth RA, Peck J, Hall P. Cone beam volume tomography: an imaging option for diagnosis of complex mandibular third molar anatomical relationships. J Calif Dent Assoc 2003;31(11):847–52.

[13] Freisfeld M, Drescher D, Kobe D, et al. Assessment of the space for the lower wisdom teeth: panoramic radiography in comparison with computed tomography. J Orofac Orthop 1998;59(1):17–28.

[14] Nakagawa Y, Kobayashi K, Ishii H, et al. Preoperative application of limited cone beam computerized tomography as an assessment tool before minor oral surgery. Int J Oral Maxillofac Surg 2002;31(3):322–6.

[15] Pawelzik J, Cohnen M, Willers R, et al. A comparison of conventional panoramic radiographs with volumetric computed tomography images in the preoperative assessment of impacted mandibular third molars. J Oral Maxillofac Surg 2002;60(9):979–84.

[16] Walters H. Reducing lingual nerve damage in third molar surgery: a clinical audit of 1350 cases. Br Dent J 1995;178(4):140–4.

[17] Mason DA. Lingual nerve damage following lower third molar surgery. Int J Oral Maxillofac Surg 1988;17(5):290–4.

[18] Pogrel MA, Goldman KE. Lingual flap retraction for third molar removal. J Oral Maxillofac Surg 2004;62(9):1125–30.

[19] Schultze-Mosgau S, Reich RH. Assessment of inferior alveolar and lingual nerve disturbances after dentoalveolar surgery, and of recovery of sensitivity. Int J Oral Maxillofac Surg 1993;22(4):214–7.

[20] Cook RT, Hutchens LH, Burkes EJ. Periodontal osseous defects associated with vitally submerged roots. J Periodontol 1977;48(5):249–60.

[21] Johnson DL, Kelly JF, Flinton RJ, et al. Histologic evaluation of vital root retention. J Oral Surg 1974; 32(11):829–33.

[22] Plata RL, Kelln EE, Linda L. Intentional retention of vital submerged roots in dogs. Oral Surg Oral Med Oral Pathol 1976;42(1):100–8.

[23] Whitaker DD, Shankle RJ. A study of the histologic reaction of submerged root segments. Oral Surg Oral Med Oral Pathol 1974;37(6):919–35.

ELSEVIER
SAUNDERS

Oral Maxillofacial Surg Clin N Am 19 (2007) 93–98

ORAL AND
MAXILLOFACIAL
SURGERY CLINICS
of North America

Risk of Periodontal Defects After Third Molar Surgery: An Exercise in Evidence-based Clinical Decision-making

Thomas B. Dodson, DMD, MPH[a,b,*],
Daniel T. Richardson, DMD, MD[b]

[a]Center of Applied Clinical Investigation, Massachusetts General Hospital, 55 Fruit Street,
Warren 1201, Boston, MA 02114, USA
[b]Departments of Oral and Maxillofacial Surgery, Harvard School of Dental Medicine,
Massachusetts General Hospital, Boston, MA, USA

The optimal management of impacted mandibular third molars (M3s) continues to challenge clinicians. An important issue to address is the risk of developing periodontal defects on the distal aspect of mandibular second molars (M2s) after M3 extraction. Kugelberg and colleagues [1–3] published several studies documenting the frequency, incidence, and risk factors for M2 periodontal pockets, such as age, inclination of M3, large contact area, visible plaque distal to M2, and pathologically widened follicle of M3, after M3 removal. For example, 2 years after M3 removal, 43.3% of the subjects had probing depths (PDs) >7 mm [1].

The purpose of this study was to apply the principles of evidence-based clinical practice to ascertain the risk for M2 periodontal defects after M3 removal. The specific aim of this study was to address the following clinical question: "Among patients having mandibular M3s removed, what is the risk of having persistent or developing new periodontal defects on the distal aspect of M2?" This question was addressed in a previous publication [4]. For this article, much of this publication is reproduced with permission of the publisher with the contents updated to incorporate more recent publications.

Materials and methods

To address the clinical question, the authors applied an evidence-based clinical practice method known as a critically appraised topic [5]. A critically appraised topic has three steps: (1) translate information needs into an answerable question, (2) identify the best evidence to answer the question, and (3) appraise the evidence for its validity (ie, its closeness to truth) and applicability (ie, usefulness in clinical practice).

Step 1: translate information needs into an answerable question

For the purpose of this article, the clinical question to answer was the following: Among patients having mandibular M3s removed, what is the risk of having persistent or developing new periodontal defects on the distal aspect of M2?

Step 2: identify the best evidence to answer the question

To find the best evidence, the authors conducted a computerized literature search of Medline using Ovid as the search engine. A summary of the search is displayed in Table 1. The resultant citations, limited to human studies and the English language, produced a candidate list of 53 studies to be reviewed in more detail.

This research activity was funded in part by a grant from the publisher and the Center for Applied Clinical Investigation in Oral and Maxillofacial Surgery.
* Corresponding author.
E-mail address: tbdodson@partners.org
(T.B. Dodson).

Table 1
Summary of literature search

	Keywords	Number of citations
1	exp[a] Molar, Third/	2788
2	limit 1 to (human and English language)	2236
3	Periodon$[b].mp.[c]	48126
4	limit 3 to (human and English language)	27744
5	Molar, third and periodont$.mp	173
6	Alveolar bone loss/	4019
7	Alveolar bone loss and molar, third	30
8	exp tooth extraction/ae [adverse effects]	2686
9	limit 8 to (human and English language)	1647
10	Tooth extraction/ae [adverse effects] and molar, third and periodon$	34
11	exp tooth, impacted/su [surgery]	1824
12	limit 11 to (human and English language)	1194
13	Tooth, impacted/su [surgery] and molar, third and periodont$.	53

[a] exp: Retrieve citations using the selected term and all of its more specific terms.

[b] $: Unlimited truncation is used to retrieve all possible suffix variations of a root word such as periodontitis, periodontal, and periodontics.

[c] mp. Ovid performs the search in fields that are customized for each database to ensure comprehensive and relevant results.

Step 3: appraise the literature

Publications considered for a more detailed review met the following inclusion criteria: (1) prospective study design, (2) follow-up data had to be available for at least 18 weeks postoperatively, (3) outcomes had to be presented in a manner that preoperative and postoperative clinical periodontal measures of attachment levels (ALs) or PDs at the distal of the M2 could be evaluated and compared. Studies with only radiographic measures of changes in alveolar bone level were excluded. Radiographic measures are indirect measures of ALs and PDs.

The key outcome variable of interest was the perioperative change (ie, preoperative versus postoperative) in AL or PD. PD was defined as the millimeter measurement from the free gingival margin to the base of the pocket. The AL was defined as the measurement in millimeters from the cemento-enamel junction to the base of the pocket. For studies that reported mean data, the preoperative and long-term follow-up measurements were compared. For the purposes of this article, clinically significant findings were defined as changes in PDs or ALs >2 mm [6].

When subject or tooth-specific data were available, periodontal status was recorded as a binary variable (ie, disease present or absent). Disease present was defined as AL >2 mm or PD >4 mm [1]. Disease absent was defined as AL ≤2 mm or PD ≤4 mm. The preoperative and postoperative disease conditions were compared using a 2 × 2 table, which permitted estimates of the treatment or harm effect of M3 removal on M2 periodontal health postoperatively.

The treatment effect or absolute risk reduction (ARR) is defined as the absolute difference between the proportion of subject with disease present pre- and postoperatively. The number needed to treat (NNT), computed as the reciprocal of ARR, is defined as the number of people with disease who must be treated to produce one positive outcome. For example, an NNT of ten suggests that ten subjects must be treated for one subject to benefit from the therapy. The smaller the NNT, the larger the therapeutic benefit of treatment.

In the setting of healthy preoperative periodontal status (ie, disease absent), there is a risk of developing periodontal defects after having M3s extracted. This risk is defined as the harm effect or the absolute risk increase (ARI). The ARI is the absolute difference between the preoperative and postoperative disease frequencies in which the postoperative disease frequency is larger than the preoperative disease frequency. The number needed to harm (NNH) is estimated by computing the reciprocal of ARI. NNH is the number of people who are treated to produce one adverse outcome. Paralleling the interpretation of NNT, an NNH of ten suggests that for every ten subjects being treated with some therapy, one subject has an adverse outcome.

Results

Ten studies met the inclusion criteria and were reviewed in detail [7–16]. Two studies were prospective cohort studies [7,10] and eight studies were randomized clinical trials [8,9,11–16]. The primary outcome of interest was change in AL or PD between the preoperative and long-term follow-up measurements.

Description of the studies

Mean data for the periodontal measures were reported in two cohort studies [7,10] and five randomized clinical trials (Table 2) [8,12,13,15,16]. Overall, when compared with preoperative measurements, PDs or ALs showed clinically insignificant changes (<2 mm) at the end of follow-up. Of note, there was one subgroup of subjects in the study reported by Ash and colleagues [7] in which the PD increased a clinically significant amount (2.4 mm) after M3 removal. This subgroup of subjects was defined as having impacted M3s that were completely covered with mucosa preoperatively.

Eight studies were randomized clinical trials designed to determine the therapeutic efficacy of reconstructing the M3 wound after extraction to enhance periodontal healing measured at M2 [8,9,11–16]. Control M3 wounds were permitted to heal spontaneously. In the setting of no measurable difference between the treatment and control groups, the results of the treatment and control groups were combined [8,9,11,12,14,15]. If there was a clinically significant treatment

Table 2
Mean data results

Study	Sample size	Age range	Outcome variables	Preoperative measurements	Postoperative measurements	Change in pre- and postoperative status
Ash et al [7]	225	14–62	AL	Completely covered M3 2.4 mm	Completely covered M3 4.7 mm	Worse[a]
				Range: 2–6 mm	Range: 2–10 mm	
				Partially covered M3 3.6 mm	Partially covered M3 3.6 mm	Unchanged
				Range: 2–7 mm	Range 2–8 mm	
				Completely erupted M3 3.0 mm	Completely erupted M3 3.4 mm	Worse[b]
				Range: 2–6	Range 2–7 mm	
Chin Quee et al [8]	30	16–30	AL	Envelope flap[e] 6.4 mm ± 0.9	Envelope flap: 6.9 mm ± 0.8	Worse[b]
				Vertical flap 6.6 mm ± 1.0	Vertical flap 7.2 mm ± 1.0	Worse[b]
Grondahl et al [10]	33	16–49	PD	4.0 mm ± 1.4[c]	2.9 mm ± 0.5	Improved[b]
Osborne et al [12]	18	18–25	PD	Control[d] 3.4 ± 0.1 mm	Control 3.6 ± 0.2 mm	Worse[b]
				Experimental 3.1 ± 0.2	Experimental 3.4 ± 0.1 mm	Worse[b]
Pecora et al [13]	10	>25	AL	Control[f] 7.4 ± 2.5 mm	Control 5.5 ± 2.4 mm	Improved[b]
Leung et al [15]	30	18–52	PD	Control 6.5 ± 1.5 mm	Control 6.7 ± 1.0 mm	Improved[a]
				Experimental 6.1 ± 1.4 mm	Experimental 2.1 ± 1.1 mm	
Sammartino et al [16]	18	21–26	PD	Control[f] 8.9 ± 0.7 mm	Control 7.2 ± 1.0 mm	Improved[b]

[a] Change in periodontal measurement was clinically significant (>2 mm).

[b] Change in periodontal measurement was clinically insignificant (≤2 mm).

[c] Mean ± standard deviation.

[d] In the experimental group, the tissue at the distal root of the M2 was planed by a periodontist, whereas on the control side neither curettage nor root planning was performed by a periodontist after M3 removal.

[e] Envelope flap was performed where the horizontal incision was brought in contact with the distal surface of the distobuccal cusp of M2. The incision continued sulcularly to the mesiobuccal line-angle of M2. The vertical flap consisted of an incision along the postmolar triangle that terminated 2 mm behind M2. The gingival collar was left intact on the distal of M2.

[f] Only data from control sites were reported, because there was evidence of a treatment effect on the experimental side.

effect, we only evaluated the control M3 sites [13,16].

When subject or tooth-specific data were available, 2×2 tables were constructed to compare the preoperative to postoperative disease status (Tables 3–7) [9,11,13,14]. Overall, 52% to 100% of the M3 sites had no change or improved disease status between the preoperative and postoperative measurements. ARR or treatment effect ranged from 10% to 41%, and the associated numbers NNTs ranged from three to ten (ie, for every three to ten M3s removed, the periodontal status of one M2 site converts from disease present preoperatively to disease absent postoperatively).

In the study by Karapataki and colleagues [11], none of the M2 sites had disease present preoperatively. In this study, the M2 periodontal health status worsened after M3 extraction in 48% of the cases. The ARI or harm effect was 48%. The associated NNH was 2. In this case, a NNH of 2 suggests that in the setting of healthy periodontium preoperatively, for every two M3s that are extracted, the periodontal status in the adjacent M2 gets worse in one case.

Discussion

The purpose of this study is to answer the question: "Among patients having their mandibular M3s extracted, what is the risk of having persistent or developing new periodontal defects on the distal aspect of the mandibular 2nd molar (M2)?" Based on the ten articles reviewed, there are two important clinical messages. First, on average, the PDs or ALs on the distal of M2 were unchanged or improved >18 weeks after M3

Table 3
Summary of binary outcomes of the periodontal status (disease present or absent) for Dodson

Postoperative status			
Preoperative	D+	D−	Total
D+	17	23	40
D−	3	5	8
Total	20	28	48

Study design: RCT split-mouth design, n = 48 M3 sites, age ≥26, AL measured.
Disease present (D+) preoperatively: 83% (40/48).
Disease present (D+) postoperatively: 42% (20/48).
Absolute risk reduction = 0.41.
Number needed to treat = 3.
Data from Dodson T. Management of mandibular 3rd molar extraction sites to prevent periodontal defects. J Oral Maxillofac Surg 2004;64:1213–24.

Table 4
Summary of binary outcomes of the periodontal status (disease present or absent) for Pecora

Postoperative status			
Preoperative	D+	D−	Total
D+	10	0	10
D−	0	0	0
Total	9	1	n = 10

Study design: RCT split-mouth design, n = 10, age ≥25, PD.
Disease present preoperatively: 100 (10/10).
Disease present postoperatively: 90% (9/10).
Absolute risk reduction = 0.10.
Number needed to treat = 10.
Data from Pecora G, Celleti R, Davapanah M, et al. The effects of guided tissue regeneration on healing after impacted mandibular third molar surgery: 1-year results. Int J Periodontol Restor Dent 1993;13:397–407.

removal. Overall, in the seven studies that reported mean data results of PD or AL, none of the studies reported clinically significant changes postoperatively [7,8,10,12,13,15,16]. In the studies in which the periodontal measures could be classified as disease present or absent, the health of the second molar improved or maintained its periodontal status between 52% and 100% of the time after M3 removal [9,11,13,14]. The NNT ranged from three to ten. For every three to ten M3s removed, the AL or PD on the distal of one adjacent M2 site improves when compared with the preoperative periodontal status.

Table 5
Summary of binary outcomes of the periodontal status (disease present or absent) for Throndson

Postoperative status			
Preoperative	D+	D−	Total
D+	3	10	13
D−	2	13	15
Total	5	23	28

Study design: RCT split-mouth design, n = 28 M3 sites, age ≥25, AL.
Disease present (D+) preoperatively (AL > 2.0 mm): 46% (13/28).
Disease present (D+) postoperatively: 18% (5/28).
Absolute risk reduction = 0.28.
Number needed to treat = 3.
Data from Throndson RR, Sexton SB. Grafting mandibular third molar extraction sites: a comparison of bioactive glass to a nongrafted site. Oral Surg Oral Med Oral Pathol 2002;94:413–9.

Table 6
Summary of binary outcomes of the periodontal status (disease present or absent) for Karapataki

Preoperative	Postoperative status		
	D+	D−	Total
D+	0	0	0
D−	19	21	40
Total	19	21	40

Study design: RCT split-mouth design, age range ≥25, n = 40 M3 sites PD or AL.

Disease present (D+) preoperatively = 0% (0/40).

Disease present (D+) postoperatively = 48% (19/40).

Absolute risk reduction = NA.

Number needed to treat = NA.

Absolute risk increase = 0.48.

Number needed to harm = 2.

Data from Karapataki S, Hugoson A, Kugelberg CF. Healing following GTR treatment of bone defects distal to mandibular 2nd molars after surgical removal of impacted 3rd molars. J Clin Periodontal 2000;27;325–32.

Second, there may be a subgroup of subjects with an increased risk for developing periodontal pockets after M3 removal (ie, subjects with healthy periodontal status preoperatively). For example, in the study by Ash and colleagues [7], in one subgroup, the completely covered M3, the PDs did worsen to a clinically significant level after M3s were removed. In the study reported by Karapataki and colleagues [11], none of the subjects had disease present preoperatively. Postoperatively, 48% of the M2 sites had converted from disease absent preoperatively to disease present postoperatively. The NNH was 2. For every two

Table 7
Summary with calculable number needed to treat and number needed to harm

Study	ARR	NNT	ARI	NNH
Dodson[a]	41%	3	N/A	N/A
Pecora et al[b]	10%	10	N/A	N/A
Throndson et al[c]	28%	3	N/A	N/A
Karapataki et al[d]	N/A	N/A	48%	2

Abbreviations: ARI, absolute risk increase; ARR, absolute risk reduction; NNH, number needed to harm; NNT, number needed to treat.

[a] Dodson: 94% had no change or improved postoperatively.

[b] Pecora et al: 100% had no change or improved postoperatively.

[c] Throndson et al: 96% had no change or improved postoperatively.

[d] Karapataki et al: 52% had no change or improved postoperatively.

healthy preoperative M2 sites, one site converts to a diseased M2 site in terms of AL or PDs after M2 removal.

Based on the results of this analysis, on average, the periodontal health on the distal of the M2 should remain unchanged or improved after M3 removal. What can be done, however, if the prognosis is in error and the periodontal measures deteriorate after M3 removal or there are clinical indications to remove M3s with healthy periodontal status? Karapataki and colleagues [17] evaluated the efficacy of guided tissue regeneration in reconstructing alveolar defects 5 years after M3 removal in sample with ALs >6 mm. The sample was composed of 20 subjects with a mean age of 43 ± 7 years. The mean preoperative and postoperative PDs were 9.5 ± 1.4 and 5.3 ± 1.9mm, respectively. The difference in PDs (4.2 mm) was clinically and statistically significant for the restorable membrane. For the nonresorbable membrane, the difference in PDs was not clinically significant.

As such, given healthy preoperative periodontal measures of PD or AL on the distal of M2, one should be circumspect in removing the M3, especially in the setting of an older subject (ie, age >25 years). In this particular study, we did not address other risk factors, such as a smoking, age, large contact area, and visible plaque distal to M2. To better ascertain the role of these other risk factors, a meta-analysis may be indicated.

Given the predictable, finite, measurable risk of bone loss after M3 surgery in subjects over the age of 25 with healthy preoperative periodontal status (ie, NNH = 2), the therapeutic indications for the operation should be articulated clearly. Alternatively, in the presence of pre-existing periodontal disease (ie, PD >4 mm or AL >2 mm), the findings of this critically appraised topic suggest that the overall periodontal health on the distal of the M2 should improve after M3 removal with NNTs ranging from three to ten.

References

[1] Kugelberg CF. Periodontal healing after impacted lower third molar surgery: a retrospective study. Int J Oral Maxillofac Surg 1985;14:29–40.

[2] Kugelberg CF, Ahlstrom U, Ericson S, et al. Periodontal healing after impacted lower third molar surgery: precision and accuracy of radiographic assessment of intrabony defects. Int J Oral Maxillofac Surg 1986;15:675–86.

[3] Kugelberg CF, Ahlstrom U, Ericson S, et al. The influence of anatomical, pathophysiological and other factors on periodontal healing after impacted lower

third molar surgery: a multiple regression analysis. J Clin Periodontol 1991;18:37–43.

[4] Richardson DT, Dodson TB. Risk of periodontal defects after third molar surgery: an exercise in evidence-based clinical decision-making. Oral Surg Oral Med Oral Pathol Oral Radiol Endod 2005; 100:133–7.

[5] Centre for Evidence-Based Medicine. The CAT bank. Available at: http://www.cebm.net/cats.asp. Accessed March 9, 2006.

[6] Greenstein G. Clinical versus Statistical significance as they relate to the efficacy of periodontal therapy. J Am Dent Assoc 2003;134:583–91.

[7] Ash M, Costich ER, Hayward R. A study of periodontal hazards of third molars. J Periodontol 1962;33:209–15.

[8] Chin Quee TA, Gosselin D, Millar EP, et al. Surgical removal of the fully impacted mandibular third molar: the influence of flap design and alveolar bone height on the periodontal status of the second molar. J Periodontol 1985;56:625–30.

[9] Dodson T. Management of mandibular 3rd molar extraction sites to prevent periodontal defects. J Oral Maxillofac Surg 2004;64:1213–24.

[10] Grondahl HG, Lekholm U. Influence of mandibular third molars on related supporting tissues. Int J Oral Maxillofac Surg 1973;2:137–42.

[11] Karapataki S, Hugoson A, Kugelberg CF. Healing following GTR treatment of bone defects distal to mandibular 2nd molars after surgical removal of impacted 3rd molars. J Clin Periodontol 2000;27: 325–32.

[12] Osborne W, Snyder A, Tempel T. Attachment levels and crevicular depths at the distal of mandibular second molars following removal of adjacent third molars. J Periodontol 1982;53:93–5.

[13] Pecora G, Celleti R, Davapanah M, et al. The effects of guided tissue regeneration on healing after impacted mandibular third -molar surgery: 1-year results. Int J Periodonontics Restorative Dent 1993;13:397–407.

[14] Throndson RR, Sexton SB. Grafting mandibular third molar extraction sites: a comparison of bioactive glass to a non-grafted site. Oral Surg Oral Med Oral Pathol 2002;94:413–9.

[15] Leung WK, Corbet EF, Kan KW, et al. A regimen of systematic periodontal care after removal of impacted mandibular third molars manages periodontal pockets associated with the mandibular second molars. J Clin Periodontol 2005;32:725–31.

[16] Sammartino G, Tia M, Marenzi G, et al. Use of autologous platelet-rich plasma (PRP) in periodontal defect treatment after extraction of impacted mandibular third molars. J Oral Maxillofac Surg 2005; 63:766–70.

[17] Karapataki S, Hugoson A, Falk H, et al. Healing following GTR treatment of intrabony defects distal to mandibular 2nd molars using resorbable and nonrestorable barriers. J Clin Periodontol 2000;27: 333–40.

ELSEVIER
SAUNDERS

Oral Maxillofacial Surg Clin N Am 19 (2007) 99–104

ORAL AND
MAXILLOFACIAL
SURGERY CLINICS
of North America

Is There a Role for Reconstructive Techniques to Prevent Periodontal Defects After Third Molar Surgery?

Thomas B. Dodson, DMD, MPH

Center of Applied Clinical Investigation, Departments of Oral and Maxillofacial Surgery, Harvard School of Dental Medicine, Massachusetts General Hospital, 55 Fruit Street, Warren 1201, Boston, MA 02114, USA

In the previous article, a comprehensive review of the literature suggests that the periodontal status on the distal of the mandibular second molar (M2) is unchanged or improved after extraction of the adjacent mandibular third molar (M3). In looking critically at the postoperative probing depths (PDs) or attachment levels (ALs), despite improvement over the preoperative condition, there still may be persistent periodontal defects. This finding begs the question: "Do other interventions need to be applied at the time of M3 removal to enhance the periodontal outcomes after M3 extraction?" Converting the information needs to an evidence-based clinical question results in the following question: "Among subjects undergoing mandibular M3 removal, does intervention at the time of tooth removal, when compared with no intervention, improve the long-term periodontal health on the distal aspect of the adjacent M2?"

A review of the literature, outlined in the previous article, identified seven randomized clinical trials (RCTs) [1–7] or prospective cohort studies [8] that help to answer the clinical question. The interventions were classified as periodontal, anatomic, or reconstructive. Periodontal interventions included mechanical débridement [3,4]. Anatomic interventions consisted of using different types of mucoperiosteal flaps to improve wound healing [1,7]. Dentoalveolar reconstructive procedures (DRPs) included guided tissue regeneration

(GTR) [5] or grafting with bone substitutes [2,8] or platelet-rich plasma (PRP) [6].

Results

Periodontal interventions

Two studies were identified that applied systematic periodontal treatment (ie, scaling and root planing) to improve the periodontal parameters (ie, PD or AL) on the distal of the mandibular M2 after M3 removal [3,4].

Osborne and colleagues [4] designed a split-mouth RCT in which subjects served as their own controls. The sample was composed of 18 subjects aged 18 to 25 years. The experimental side received preoperative curettage and root planing. The control side received no treatment. The outcome variable was PD measured preoperatively and 12 months postoperatively. Preoperatively, the PDs for the control and experimental sides were 3.4 and 3.1 mm, respectively, which suggested minimal disease present preoperatively. At 1 year postoperatively, the PDs had increased in both groups by <1 mm and there was no statistically significant difference between the two treatment groups (0.1 mm; $P > 0.05$).

Leung and colleagues [3] designed an RCT and a sample of 30 subjects who completed follow-up and had a mean age of 32 years, mesioangular impactions, and pre-existing periodontal defects (PD >5 mm). One M3 per subject was used. The sample was randomized into two groups: control and experimental. The control group had standard socket débridement after M3 removal. The experimental group had standard socket débridement after M3 removal, and the M2 underwent

This research activity was funded in part by a grant from the publisher and the Center for Applied Clinical Investigation in Oral and Maxillofacial Surgery.

E-mail address: tbdodson@partners.org

Table 1
Summary of the articles

Author	Treatment category	Risk factors[a]	Study design	Sample size	Treatment control	Outcome variable	Preoperative findings	Postoperative findings	Change	P values
Osborne et al [4]	Periodontal	None	RCT, split-mouth	18	Periodontal therapy	PDs measured preoperatively and 12 months postoperatively	3.1 ± 0.2	3.4 ± 0.1	−0.3	$P > 0.05$
					No treatment		3.4 ± 0.1	3.6 ± 0.2	−0.2	$P > 0.05$
Leung et al [3]	Periodontal	Age, periodontal status, tooth position	RCT	14 Tx	Periodontal therapy	PDs (mm) measured preoperatively and 6 months postoperatively	6.1 ± 1.4	2.1 ± 1.1	4 mm	<0.01
				16 Cntl	No treatment		6.5 ± 1.5	2.7 ± 1.0	3.8 mm	<0.01
Stephens et al [7]	Anatomic	None	RCT, split-mouth	15	Envelope with distal wedge	PDs (mm) measured preoperatively and 12 weeks postoperatively	NR	NR	1.9	0.001
					Envelope with distal wedge and vertical release				2.0	<0.001
Chin Quee et al [1]	Anatomic	None	RCT, split-mouth	25	Envelope flap with vertical release	AL measured preoperatively and 6 months postoperatively	6.6 ± 1.0	7.2 ± 1.0	−0.6 mm	<0.001
					Envelope flap without release		6.4 ± 0.9	6.9 ± 0.8	−0.5 mm	<0.001

Study		Design	Adjusted for	N	Treatment	Outcome				P value
Dodson [2]	DRP	RCT, split-mouth	Age	12	DBP	PDs[b] measured preoperatively and 26 weeks postoperatively	7.3 ± 3.5	3.7 ± 1.6	3.6 ± 3.6	0.005
Pecora et al [5]	DRP	RCT	Age, periodontal status, tooth position	12	GTR	AL measured preoperatively and 12 months postoperatively	6.2 ± 2.3	4.3 ± 1.4	1.9 ± 3.1	0.053
				24	No tx		6.7 ± 2.6	4.1 ± 1.5	2.6 ± 2.5	<0.001
				10	GTR		7.5 ± 2.9	3.2 ± 1.0	4.3 ± 2.5	<0.01
Dodson [8]	DRP	Cohort	Age, periodontal status, tooth position	10	No tx	AL measured preoperatively and 26 weeks postoperatively	7.4 ± 2.5	5.5 ± 2.4	1.9 ± 1.7	<0.01
				5	DBP		7.6 ± 3.5	1.4 ± 0.5	6.2 ± 3.3	0.014
Sammartino [6]	DRP	RCT, split-mouth	Periodontal status tooth position	5	GTR	PDs measured preoperatively and 12 weeks postoperatively	5.4 ± 2.1	3.0 ± 1.2	2.4 ± 3.0	0.15
				8	No tx		6.8 ± 2.3	3.8 ± 0.9	3.0 ± 2.9	0.023
				18	PRP		8.9 ± 1.0	3.7 ± 1.3	5.4 mm	<0.01
					No tx		8.9 ± 0.7	7.2 ± 1.7	1.7	<0.05

Abbreviations: AL, attachment level; DBP, demineralized bone powder; DRP, dentoalveolar reconstructive procedure; GTR, guided tissue regeneration; NR, not reported; PD, probing depths.

[a] Age >25, pre-existing periodontal disease, tooth position.

[b] For brevity, only PD is reported in this table. Both PD and AL were recorded and results were similar.

ultrasonic root débridement followed by a three-visit plaque control program. PDs were measured preoperatively and over time for 6 months after M3 removal. There were 16 and 14 subjects in the control and treatment groups, respectively. There was a statistically and clinically significant improvement in terms of PDs in the control (3.8 mm; $P < 0.01$) and treatment (4.0 mm; $P < 0.01$) groups, but there was no clinically or statistically significant difference between the two treatment groups (0.2 mm; $P > 0.05$).

Anatomic interventions

Two studies were identified by applying different types of mucoperiosteal flap designs to improve the periodontal measures on the distal of the mandibular M2 after M3 removal [1,7].

Stephens and colleagues [7] implemented an RCT and enrolled a sample of 15 subjects aged 20 to 26 who needed extraction of two mandibular M3s. The predictor variable was the type of incision used to access the M3 (ie, envelope with distal wedge [conventional] or envelope with distal wedge and a release [experimental]). The study was designed as a split-mouth model with subjects serving as their own controls. The outcome variable was PD measured preoperatively and at 2, 6, and 12 weeks postoperatively. Probing depths were measured at the distal, distobuccal, and facial of the M2. For the purposes of this analysis, the author of this article selected one landmark: distobuccal [2]. Having multiple landmarks to analyze creates a challenging analytic problem, and the interpretation of the results is difficult at best. Briefly, when compared with the preoperative measurement, the PDs for both incisions improved by approximately 2 mm when measured 12 weeks after M3 extraction ($P < 0.03$) and there was no difference between the two incision types (0.1 mm; $P > 0.05$) (Table 1).

Chin Quee and colleagues [1] implemented a split-mouth RCT and enrolled a sample of 25 subjects aged 16 to 30 who required extraction of bilateral mandibular M3s and completed follow-up. The M3s to be extracted were randomly assigned to be accessed via a vertical or envelope flap. The ALs were measured preoperatively and 6 months postoperatively. There was a statistically but nonclinically significant difference in ALs in both treatment groups (-0.5 mm) over time. The difference between treatment groups, however, was not clinically or statistically significant (0.1 mm; $P > 0.05$).

Dentoalveolar reconstructive procedures

Four studies applied DRPs (ie, GTR) [5], bone substitutes (demineralized bone powder [DBP]) [2,8], and PRP [6] to enhance postoperative periodontal measures on the distal of the mandibular M2 after extracting the adjacent M2.

Dodson [2] implemented a split-mouth RCT and enrolled a sample of 24 subjects age ≥ 26 years. Subjects were randomly assigned to one of two treatment groups: DBP or resorbable GTR. These materials were used to reconstruct the M3 extraction site at the time of M3 removal. Subjects served as their own controls. Within each subject, treatment and control sides were randomly assigned. On the control site, the M3 extraction site was debrided, irrigated, and closed primarily. The outcome variables were PD and AL measured preoperatively and 26 weeks after extraction. For the purposes of this article, only PD is reported, but the results are similar for AL. In all three groups (ie, DBP, GTR, and control), the PDs improved over time. In the DBP and control groups, the improvements were clinically and statistically significant (Table 1). In the GTR group, the change was near clinically and statistically significant. There were, however, no clinically or statistically significant differences among the three groups, which suggested no benefit to treatment over control. There also was a statistically significant increased risk of inflammatory complications in the treatment M3s compared with the control M3s ($P = 0.049$). The results of this study that suggest neither DBP nor GTR offered a predictable benefit over no treatment. Given the increased risk of postoperative inflammatory complications in the treatment group, these reconstructive materials are not indicated for routine use after M3 removal.

Kugelberg and colleagues [9] applied a multifactorial approach to identify predictors of postoperative intrabony defects on the distal of M2 after M3 removal. The sample consisted of 144 subjects having 215 mandibular M3s removed. The investigators identified three types of variables associated with an increased risk for periodontal defects after M3 surgery. These factors were age > 25 years, preoperative periodontal defect (AL ≥ 4 mm), and close proximity between the distal of the M2 and M3 as evidenced by a mesioangular or horizontal impaction, root resorption of the M2, or an enlarged M3 follicle.

Pecora and colleagues [5] designed a RCT and enrolled a sample of 20 subjects who had three risk factors for adverse periodontal outcomes after M3 surgery as outlined by Kugelberg And colleagues [9] To be enrolled in the sample, the subjects were >26 years of age, had horizontally impacted M3s, and had PDs ≥5 mm. Subjects were randomly assigned to a test or control group. In the test group, the M3 site was reconstructed using GTR (nonresorbable). In the control group, no treatment was rendered other than débridement of the socket. In both groups, there was a statistically significant improvement in ALs 1 year after M3 extraction. In the treatment group, the improvement was clinically significant, 4.3 ± 2.5 mm. In the control group, the improvement was near clinically significant, 1.9 ± 1.7 mm. The difference between the two treatment groups, 2.4 mm, was clinically and statistically significant ($P < 0.01$). These findings suggest that in the setting of a high-risk subject, that GTR may be indicated to limit the risk of developing a periodontal defect after M3 removal.

Dodson [8] reviewed the study sample enrolled in the RCT summarized previously and was able to identify a cohort of subjects who had M3s that could be considered high risk for developing periodontal defects after M3 removal (ie, age ≥26 years, mesioangular or horizontal impaction, and a pre-existing AL ≥3 mm) [9]. The sample was composed of 12 subjects with 18 high-risk M3s. There were 8 control M3s, 5 M3 extraction sites reconstructed with GTR, and 5 M3 extraction sites reconstructed with DBP. All three types of extractions sites demonstrated clinically significant improvement in ALs (>2 mm), but only the control and DBP treated groups reach statistical significance ($P < 0.05$). The M3s sites treated with DBP had clinically and statistically significantly improved ALs when compared with the control and GTR treated sites, $P = 0.001$ and 0.037, respectively. The control and GTR sites were neither clinically or statistically significantly different. These findings suggest that subjects at high risk for developing M2 periodontal defects after M3 surgery may benefit from the use of DBP placed at the time of M3 removal to improve postoperative periodontal healing on the distal of the M2.

Sammartino and colleagues [6] implemented a split-mouth RCT and enrolled a sample of 18 subjects (aged 21–26) with pre-existing periodontal defects (PD ≥7.5 mm) and mesioangular impactions who required extraction of two mandibular M3s. This sample has two of the three factors associated with high-risk M3 extraction sites. The M3 selected for treatment was reconstructed with PRP placed into the extraction wound after M3 removal and scaling and root planing of the distal root surface of the adjacent M2 The control side had the M3 wound débrided and distal of the adjacent M2 was scaled and root planned. PDs were measured preoperatively and 18 weeks postoperatively. At 18 weeks postoperatively, there was a statistically significant improvement in PDs in the control and treatment groups, 1.7 and 5.4 mm, respectively. The treatment group had a clinically and statistically significant improvement in PDs over the control group.

Summary

The purpose of this article is to address the following clinical question: "Among subjects undergoing mandibular M3 removal, does an intervention at the time of tooth removal, when compared with no intervention, improve the long-term periodontal health on the distal aspect of the adjacent M2?"

In brief, routine application of interventions to improve the periodontal parameters on the distal of the M2 at the time of M3 removal is not indicated for all subjects. There seems to be a subpopulation of subjects having M3s removed who are at increased risk for periodontal defects after M3 removal (ie, age ≥26 years, pre-existing periodontal defects [AL ≥3 mm or PDs ≥5 mm], and a horizontal or mesioangular impaction). In the setting of having all three risk factors present, there seems to be a predictable benefit to treating the dentoalveolar defect at the time of extraction. Although nonresorbable GTR, DBP, and PRP all work well in the setting of high-risk M3s, DBP is the simplest and most inexpensive to use. In the author's practice, having patients with all three risk factors present is an uncommon event (<20 cases per year). When the risk factors are present, the author recommends grafting the M3 extraction site with DBP. Generally, 2 cc of DBP is adequate to fill the defect. The wound is closed primarily with a resorbable suture and the patient is placed on an antibacterial mouth rinse and a short course of oral antibiotics (eg, penicillin) for 5 to 7 days. The efficacy of the mouth rinse or antibiotics is unknown.

References

[1] Chin Quee TA, Gosselin D, Millar EP, et al. Surgical removal of the fully impacted mandibular third molar: the influence of flap design and alveolar bone

height on the periodontal status of the second molar.
J Periodontal 1985;56:625–30.

[2] Dodson TB. Management of 3rd molar extraction
sites to prevent periodontal defects. J Oral Maxillofac
Surg 2004;62:1213–24.

[3] Leung WK, Corbet EF, Kan KW, et al. A regimen of
systematic periodontal care after removal of impacted
mandibular third molars manages periodontal
pockets associated with the mandibular second
molars. J Clin Periodontol 2005;32:725–31.

[4] Osborne WH, Snyder AJ, Tempel TR. Attachment
levels and crevicular depths at the distal of mandibular second molars following removal of adjacent third
molars. J Periodontol 1982;53(2):93–5.

[5] Pecora G, Celleti R, Davapanah M, et al. The effects
of guided tissue regeneration on healing after impacted mandibular third molar surgery: 1-year results.
Int J Periodontics Restorative Dent 1993;13:397–407.

[6] Sammartino G, Tia M, Marenzi G, et al. Use of autologous platelet-rich plasma (PRP) in periodontal
defect treatment after extraction of impacted
mandibular third molars. J Oral Maxillofac Surg
2005;63:766–70.

[7] Stephens RJ, App GR, Foreman DW. Periodontal
evaluation of two mucoperiosteal flaps used in
removing impacted mandibular third molars. J Oral
Maxillofac Surg 1983;41:719–24.

[8] Dodson TB. Is there a role for reconstructive
techniques to prevent periodontal defects after
third molar surgery. J Oral Maxillofac Surg 2005;
63:891.

[9] Kugelberg CF, Ahlstrom U, Ericson S, et al. The
influence of anatomical, pathophysiological and
other factors on periodontal healing after impacted
lower third molar surgery: a multiple regression
analysis. J Clin Periodontol 1991;18:37–43.

ELSEVIER
SAUNDERS

Oral Maxillofacial Surg Clin N Am 19 (2007) 105–115

ORAL AND
MAXILLOFACIAL
SURGERY CLINICS
of North America

Nerve Injuries After Third Molar Removal

Vincent B. Ziccardi, DDS, MD[a,*], John R. Zuniga, DMD, MS, PhD[b]

[a]Department of Oral and Maxillofacial Surgery, University of Medicine and Dentistry of New Jersey,
110 Bergen Street, Room B-854, Newark, NJ 07103-2400, USA
[b]Division of Oral and Maxillofacial Surgery, University of Texas Medical Center, 5323 Harry Hines Boulevard,
Dallas, TX 75390-9109, USA

The peripheral branches of the trigeminal nerve are susceptible to injury from the surgical removal of third molars. These injuries can be devastating for patients because of their effects on speech, mastication, swallowing, and social interactions. Fortunately, most of these trigeminal nerve injuries undergo spontaneous recovery. Some injuries may be permanent, however, with varying outcomes ranging from mild hypoesthesia to complete paresthesia and neuropathic responses resulting in chronic pain syndromes [1].

The face and perioral region have a high density of peripheral nerve receptors, which makes it unpleasant for patients to tolerate or adapt to neurosensory disturbances. Pain, temperature, and proprioception are transmitted centrally through the lingual, mental, inferior alveolar, infraorbital, and supraorbital nerves. Each of these sensory modalities must be evaluated in the neurosensory assessment of patients and monitored for recovery postoperatively [2]. The goal of trigeminal microsurgery is to create an environment in which those nerves thought not to be susceptible for spontaneous recovery are given the best opportunity for regeneration. This article discusses patient assessment, microsurgical treatments, and outcome assessments for patients who sustain inferior alveolar nerve (IAN) and lingual nerve injuries from third molar removal.

The complications and expected postoperative sequelae that result from the surgical removal of third molar removal are well documented. Most patients report some degree of pain, bleeding, swelling, trismus, bruising, and stretching of the lips, especially the area of the oral commissure. Temporary or permanent sensory nerve disturbances are not uncommon; however, the incidence of lingual and IAN injuries reported ranges from 0.4% to 22%. Sensory deficits that last longer than 1 year are likely to be permanent, and attempts for microsurgical repair are often unpredictable after that time. Surgeons must be aware of this complication and provide detailed preoperative informed consent to their patients [3,4].

The incidence of neurologic injuries from third molar surgery may be related to multiple factors, including surgeon experience and proximity of the tooth relative to the IAN canal. Horizontally impacted teeth are generally more difficult to remove because of the increased need for bone removal and soft tissue manipulation when compared with distoangular or mesioangular impactions with a higher incidence of nerve injuries [5]. Third molar surgery performed under general anesthesia compared with surgery performed under local anesthesia has been reported to have a higher incidence of nerve injuries, presumably because of the supine position of the patient and extent of soft tissue dissection, potential greater surgical forces that may be applied under general anesthesia, and overall more difficult surgical case selection [6]. Other studies have found no significant relationship between nerve injury and the anesthetic modality [7].

IAN injury secondary to third molar removal also has been correlated with patient age over 35 and the presence of completely developed roots.

* Corresponding author.
  E-mail address: ziccarvb@umdnj.edu (V.B. Ziccardi).

The depth of impaction and the degree of imposition of the root structures over the inferior alveolar canal space have been found to contribute to an increased incidence of postoperative nerve injuries. The use of rotary instrumentation and surgical sectioning of teeth with exposure of the mandibular canal also can be associated with sensory nerve disturbances. Teeth with one large root requiring buccal bone removal with rotary instrumentation, however, have been associated with a higher incidence of lingual nerve injuries [8]. Consideration may be given for the use of intentional partial odontectomy in patients thought to be at high risk for potential nerve injuries provided no pathologic condition is present.

Lingual nerve injuries that result from third molar surgery have been reported to occur in 0.5% to 22% of all patients. Patients with lingual nerve injury report drooling, tongue biting, thermal burns, changes in speech, and swallowing and taste perception alterations. Because of the potentially varied anatomic position of the lingual nerve, the surgeon is not always able to identify its location. Studies have described the position of the lingual nerve using cadaveric dissections and MRI to lie above the lingual crest in 10% of patients and even in direct contact with the lingual plate in up to 25% of patients [9,10]. Any surgical incisions placed too far lingually or breaching the lingual cortex with a surgical bur may jeopardize the lingual nerve. Other anatomic factors, such as lingual angulation of the third molar, need for vertical sectioning, prolonged operating time, and surgeon inexperience, have been found to increase the risk for lingual nerve injury [11]. The use of lingual flap retraction during third molar surgery has been associated with an increased incidence of transient sensory disturbances; however, it is neither protective nor detrimental in regards to permanent lingual nerve injury [12].

Classification of trigeminal nerve injuries

Seddon [13] and Sunderland [14] developed classification systems for nerve injuries based on the degree of nerve disruption that are still useful currently (Table 1). These systems were based on the degree of injury affecting the endoneurium, perineurium, epineurium, and supporting tissues. Seddon's classification is based on the time from injury and degree of observed sensory recovery, whereas the Sunderland classification emphasizes the fascicular structure of the nerve and the

amount of nerve damage [15]. Seddon proposed three categories of nerve injury, including neuropraxia, axonotmesis, and neurotmesis. Sunderland expanded the Seddon classification to include five degrees of nerve injury.

Neuropraxia (Sunderland first-degree injury) results from minor compression or traction of the nerve trunk, which results in a conduction blockade. Axonal continuity is maintained, which results in a temporary conduction blockade. Significant traction injuries may result in vascular stasis with focal neural demyelination. Patients clinically report sensory disturbances lasting from hours to months, depending on the severity of injury with complete recovery. Trigeminal microsurgery is not indicated unless a foreign body is present, which would be an indication for microsurgery.

Axonotmesis (Sunderland second-degree injury) is produced by crush or significant traction injuries. These injuries are similar to first-degree injuries with some degree of Wallerian degeneration distal to the zone of injury. There is no degeneration of the endoneurium, perineurium, or epineurium, which allows for the axons to regenerate. Sensory recovery is usually complete in 2 to 4 months but may take up to 1 year for complete recovery. Trigeminal nerve microsurgery is not indicated unless a foreign body is impeding nerve regeneration.

Third- and fourth-degree Sunderland injuries do not have a corresponding Seddon category. Third-degree injuries result from moderate to severe crushing or traction of the nerve. Wallerian degeneration is present, with some neuron death occurring. Disruption of the endoneurium does not allow complete regeneration of the axon, which results in mild to moderate permanent sensory nerve disturbances. Trigeminal nerve microsurgery may be indicated if there is no sensory nerve recovery after 3 months. No absolute optimal time for repair of trigeminal nerve injuries has been established.

Fourth-degree Sunderland injuries occur with endoneural and perineural disruption and result in permanent alteration of the blood-nerve barrier. Neuronal loss occurs with the possibility of neuroma formation. Intraneural scars and fibrosis also may develop, which can further impede the process of regeneration. An increase in the intraneural pressure contributes to degeneration and adversely affects the prognosis for recovery. Microsurgical intervention is indicated if there is no significant sensory recovery by 3 or more months.

Table 1
Seddon and Sunderland classification of nerve injuries

Injury classification	Cause	Healing	Microsurgery
Neuropraxia (Seddon) First-degree injury (Sunderland)	Minor nerve compression or traction injury	Spontaneous recovery in less than 2 months	Not indicated unless foreign body impeding nerve regeneration
Axonotmesis (Seddon) Second-degree injury (Sunderland)	Crush or traction injury	Spontaneous recovery in 2–4 months Up to 1 year for complete recovery	Not indicated unless foreign body present
Third-degree injury (Sunderland)	Traction, compression, or crush injury	Some spontaneous recovery, but not complete	Microsurgery indicated if no improvement by 3 months
Fourth-degree injury (Sunderland)	Traction, compression, injection, or chemical injury	Poor prognosis for spontaneous recovery High probability for neuroma formation or intraneural fibrosis	Microsurgery indicated if no significant improvement after 3 months
Neurotmesis (Seddon) Fifth-degree injury (Sunderland)	Transection, avulsion, or laceration of nerve trunk	Poor prognosis Extensive fibrosis, neuroma formation, or neuropathic changes	Microsurgery indicated if no improvement after 3 months or development of neuropathic response

Neurotmesis (Sunderland fifth-degree injury) is characterized by complete transection of the nerve trunk affecting all layers of the nerve. This injury results in complete disruption of the nerve with possible neuroma formation and poor prognosis for spontaneous recovery. These lesions clinically demonstrate complete anesthesia of the affected target area with the potential for the development of neuropathic responses. Trigeminal microsurgery is definitely indicated for this group of injuries.

Clinical neurosensory testing

Neurosensory testing should be performed to determine the degree of sensory impairment, monitor recovery, and determine whether trigeminal nerve microsurgery is indicated. Clinical neurosensory testing can be divided into mechanoceptive and nociceptive testing based on the specific receptor stimulated. Mechanoceptive testing includes two-point discrimination, static light touch, brush stroke, and vibrational sense. Nociceptive testing includes pain stimuli and thermal discrimination. Mechanoceptive testing should be completed before nociceptive testing. Testing should be performed in a reproducible manner

with the patient seated comfortably in a semi-reclined and comfortable position. The affected area is first mapped using the directional brush stroke to discern normal from abnormal areas. This procedure may be accomplished by marking directly on the patient's skin and photographing the area for documentation or recording on a standardized testing form. Mapping is used to delineate the area where testing should be performed.

Static light touch is assessed using the Von Frey monofilaments, which are calibrated with the log base ten of the magnitude of force in milligrams required to bend the filament, which evaluates the A-beta fibers and pressure perception. The monofilament is applied perpendicular to the skin and pressure is applied just until the filament begins to bend in sequential order until the patient can perceive the sensation. For the trigeminal nerve, detection of the 1.65 to 2.36 monofilament is considered normal for static light touch. If the Von Frey monofilaments are not available, a crude approximation of static light touch is achieved by using a wisp of cotton to stroke the skin gently to determine sensory perception.

Two-point discrimination can be tested using an ECG caliper, boley gauge, or two-point anesthesiometer. The test is performed and re-peated in 2-mm increments until the patient can no longer perceive two distinct points. The boley gauge is useful for this purpose because it is readily available and accurate to within 1 mm. Normal values for the inferior alveolar and lingual nerve distributions are approximately 4 mm and 3 mm, respectively. Values more than 20 mm are not recorded because it would measure sensation from the contralateral zone of innervation.

Brush directional discrimination is assessed using a fine hairbrush or the baseline Von Frey monofilament used for the static light touch. This test assesses the integrity of the large myelinated A-alpha and A-beta fibers. The brush is stroked across the skin in a 1-cm area and the patient is asked whether he or she perceives the sensation and the direction of the stroke. The patient should be able to perceive the stroke sensation and travel direction in at least 90% of the application for a normal result.

Pin pressure nociception assesses the free nerve endings innervated by the lightly myelinated A-delta and unmyelinated C-fibers. This test is simply performed by using a sterile dental needle, which is applied in a quick prick fashion in sufficient intensity to be perceived by the patient. Appropriate response would be the perception of sharp and not just pressure. Alternatively, a pressure algesiometer may be used to consistently provide a standardized amount of pressure, usually 25 g.

Thermal discrimination can be performed using a cotton applicator sprayed with ethyl chloride for the perception of cold, which is mediated by the unmyelinated C-fibers. Heat perception is transmitted by the A-delta fiber, which may be tested using heated gutta percha. Minnesota thermal discs also may be used to test for thermal discrimination.

Diagnostic nerve blocks can be a useful adjunct in the assessment of patients who have pain as a presenting symptom. The purpose of diagnostic nerve blocks is to isolate the affected region of the nerve and determine what level of fiber is affected. Dilute local anesthetic agents can block the small nerve fibers, whereas higher concentrations are required to block the larger myelinated fibers. These blocks are usually initiated at the periphery and then administered centrally along trigeminal nerve pathways. Ineffective nerve blocks may indicate either that the nerve was not appropriately blocked or that

collateral macrosprouting has developed from adjacent nerves. If diagnostic nerve blocks are effective in relieving pain, microsurgery may be indicated. Patients who experience no relief from diagnostic nerve blocks may have a centrally mediated pain syndrome, which would be a contraindication for trigeminal microsurgery and consideration for pharmacologic management.

Zuniga and colleagues [16] demonstrated that clinical neurosensory testing is a reliable diagnostic tool in evaluating lingual nerve injuries based on preoperative testing compared with actual intraoperative findings from trigeminal microsurgery. For inferior alveolar injuries, they reported that clinical neurosensory testing was useful for ruling in IAN injuries but less reliable for ruling out inferior alveolar injuries. Based on these findings, they concluded that clinician also must consider other factors, such as patient age, mechanism of injury, time since injury, and the presence of neuropathic pain regarding indications for trigeminal nerve microsurgery.

Indications for trigeminal nerve microsurgery

If symptoms of nerve injury persist for more than 3 months with no improvement, microsurgical intervention may be considered. Indications for trigeminal nerve microsurgery include (1) observed nerve transection, (2) no improvement in hypoesthesia for 3 months, (3) development of pain caused by nerve entrapment or neuroma formation, (4) presence of a foreign body, (5) progressively worsening hypoesthesia or dysesthesia, and (6) hypoesthesia that is intolerable to the patient. Contraindications for trigeminal microsurgery include (1) central neuropathic pain, (2) evidence of improving sensory function, (3) hypoesthesia that is acceptable to the patient, (4) metabolic neuropathy, (5) severely medically compromised patient, (6) extremes of age, and (7) excessive time since injury.

Nerve repairs are categorized as primary, delayed primary, and secondary depending on their timing relative to the initial injury. Primary nerve repairs are performed immediately at the time of an observed injury. If a surgeon is not proficient in trigeminal microsurgery, these patients may be sent to a microsurgeon who could perform the repair within a few weeks for a delayed primary repair. Unobserved injuries, which are the most common, are injuries that present to the surgeon after surgery has been completed.

These patients should undergo serial neurosensory examinations and be considered as microsurgical candidates based on the previously mentioned criteria.

Trigeminal nerve microsurgery

Trigeminal microsurgery generally should be performed before 1 year if reinnervation of distal end organs is to be expected. Significant distal nerve scarring and atrophy occur by 1 year, which makes microsurgery less predictable. Microsurgery is best performed in the operating room under general anesthesia with complete muscle relaxation. The operating room table is turned 90° relative to the anesthesiologist to allow for placement of the surgical microscope. Repair may be performed using surgical loupes; however, an operating microscope with multiple heads allows the surgeon and assistant simultaneous views of the surgical field (Fig. 1). Instrumentation for trigeminal nerve microsurgery minimally consists of microforceps, scissors, needle holders, and nerve hooks. A beaver blade is useful for internal dissection and preparation of the nerve for neurorrhaphy or excision of scar tissue.

Basic surgical principles for trigeminal nerve microsurgery include exposure, hemostasis, visualization, removal of scar tissue, nerve preparation, and nerve anastomosis without tension. Clotted blood in proximity to a nerve repair may increase the amount of connective tissue proliferation and lead to further extrinsic scarring and compression-induced ischemia, creating possible demyelination and reduced sensory recovery. Hemostasis can be enhanced with the use of reverse Trendelenberg position, hypotensive anesthetic techniques, and local anesthesia with vasoconstrictor. Bone bleeding may be controlled through use of bone wax or other hemostatic agents. Electocoagulation is facilitated using bipolar cautery to minimize collateral injury to the nerve.

A transoral approach is most commonly used for trigeminal microneurosurgery. Exposure of the IAN can be accomplished after decorticating the lateral cortex through a vestibular incision. Alternatively, a cutaneous incision placed in a resting skin line may be indicated for cases in which the area of injury is not readily accessible by an intraoral approach. The lingual nerve is approached through either a paralingual or lingual gingival sulcus incision. The paralingual mucosal incision is completed with blunt and sharp dissection to expose the nerve. Advantages of the paralingual approach include use of a smaller incision with direct visualization; however, transected nerve ends may retract from the surgical field on blunt dissection. The lingual gingival sulcus incision requires a lateral release along the external oblique ridge for complete flap mobilization. The nerve is visualized from below the periosteum once the flap is elevated, which allows the nerve to be dissected bluntly from the flap. This technique requires a larger incision than

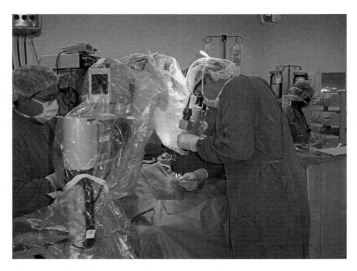

Fig. 1. Use of multiple head operating microscope for trigeminal nerve microsurgery.

the paralingual mucosal incision design; however, the proximal and distal nerve ends do not retract from the field during dissection (Figs. 2 and 3) [17].

External neurolysis is the surgical procedure to free the nerve from its tissue bed and remove any restrictive scar tissue or bone in the case of IAN injuries. Damage to soft tissues surrounding a nerve may result in scar tissue formation and create a compressive entrapment-type injury. External neurolysis is generally performed under some magnification to grossly assess the nerve and isolate any physical abnormalities [18]. For some patients, external neurolysis may be the only surgical procedure indicated. Once the external neurolysis is completed, the nerve is examined under magnification and intraoperative findings dictate any additional procedures. Foreign bodies, such as endodontic filling material, tooth fragments, or implant materials, should be removed at this point.

Internal neurolysis is indicated when there is evidence of nerve fibrosis or gross changes in the external appearance of the nerve. This procedure requires the opening of the epineurium to examine the internal fascicular structure of the nerve. Because the trigeminal nerve has a sparse amount of epineurium, any manipulation potentially can lead to further scar tissue formation. Therefore, some surgeons question the use of this procedure. The procedure begins with the elevation of the epineurium facilitated through the injection of saline within the affected nerve segment. A longitudinal incision is made through the epineurium using a beaver blade to expose the internal structures in a procedure referred to as an epifascicular epineurotomy. With release of the epineural fibrosis, the nerve may expand, which indicates a successful internal neurolysis procedure. A circumferential portion of the epineurium may be removed in a procedure called epifascicular epineurectomy. If no expansion is noted and complete fibrosis is observed, the affected segment should be excised and the nerve prepared for primary neurorrhaphy.

Excision of neuromas is performed to allow for reanastomosis of complete nerve injuries in an effort to re-establish continuity and allow for nerve regeneration. After excision of the neuroma or nonviable nerve tissue, the resulting segments are examined under magnification to ascertain whether normal tissue is present, which is determined by the presence of herniated intrafascicular tissues. The goal is to allow the suturing of the two nerve ends together without tension in a process called primary neurorrhaphy. The two nerve segments are approximated using 7-0 or smaller nonreactive epineural sutures. This portion of the procedure is completed using microinstrumentation under magnification. Mobilization of the IAN may be augmented by distal and proximal nerve dissection or sacrifice of the incisive branch of the IAN, which requires decortication of the IAN from the site of injury to the mental foramina (Figs. 4–6). This manipulation may allow up to an additional 10 mm of mobilization to facilitate tension-free nerve repairs [19]. Regardless of the suture technique selected, tension across the nerve repair must be minimized. Tension more than 25 g has been demonstrated to have a deleterious effect on nerve regeneration because of gapping and formation of scar tissue, which may inhibit axon proliferation through the site of repair [20].

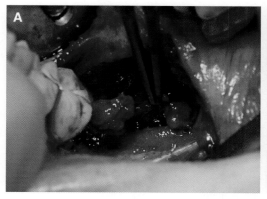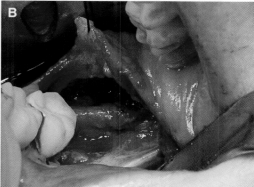

Fig. 2. (*A*) Intraoperative view depicts proximal and distal lingual nerve before preparation for neurorrhaphy. (*B*) Lingual nerve after primary neurorrhaphy.

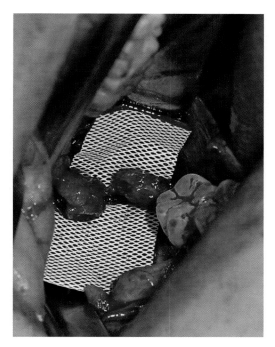

Fig. 3. Intraoperative photograph of a complete lingual nerve injury before preparation for repair.

Nerve grafts

The primary indication for trigeminal nerve grafting involves cases that result in a continuity defect that cannot be repaired primarily or without excessive tension. The selection of a donor site for interpositional nerve grafting is predicated on several factors, such as nerve diameter and fascicular pattern, correlation of neural function

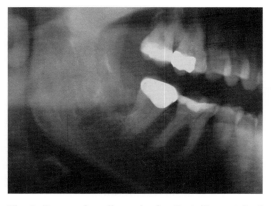

Fig. 4. Panoramic radiograph of patient who sustained IAN injury after third molar removal. Note the superimposition of the third molar roots over the IAN canal shadow.

(eg, sensory or motor), ease of graft procurement, and potential donor site morbidity. For trigeminal nerve repairs, the sural and greater auricular nerves meet most of these requirements, including ease of procurement and relatively tolerable resultant donor site anesthesia [21].

Diameter of the donor nerve graft should correlate with the diameter of the host nerve. The IAN averages approximately 2.4 mm diameter and the lingual nerve 3.2 mm diameter. The sural nerve is approximately 2.1 mm in diameter and the greater auricular nerve averages 1.5 mm diameter; thus, there is no exact match available for trigeminal nerve grafting. Cross-sectional shape of the IAN and lingual nerves is generally round, whereas the sural nerve is flat and the greater auricular nerve is oval.

The fascicular number and size of fascicles should correspond between the donor and recipient sites. The IAN has between 18 and 21 fascicles in the third molar region, which decreases to approximately 12 fascicles at the mental nerve, whereas the lingual nerve commonly has between 15 and 18 fascicles in the third molar region and more at the distal termination. The sural nerve generally provides 11 to 12 fascicles, and the greater auricular nerve usually has 8 or 9 fascicles as a single graft. Pogrel and colleagues [22] reported that the lingual nerve had a mean of 3 fascicles (range 1–8) at the level of the lingula and a mean of 20 fascicles (range 7–39) at the third molar region. Four specimens were monofascicular at the level of the lingula. The IAN had a mean of 7.2 fascicles (range 3–14) at the level of the lingula. In all cases, the lingual nerve had the same number or fewer fascicles than the IAN at the level of the lingula. Because of the smaller fascicular size and overall nerve diameter, the sural nerve graft precludes direct fascicular alignment, but chance apposition of the fascicular cross-section at the suture line allows passage of regenerative axonal sprouts. This effect is enhanced by the sparse epineurium present within the trigeminal nerve [23]. The final consideration in nerve graft procurement is donor site morbidity. The sural nerve graft results in numbness over the heel and lateral aspect of the foot, whereas the greater auricular nerve harvest results in numbness to the lateral neck, skin overlying the posterior mandible, and the ear [24].

Several other materials have been proposed for nerve grafting, including alloplastic tubules, skeletal muscle, and vein grafts. The technique of entubilization using alloplastic materials is an

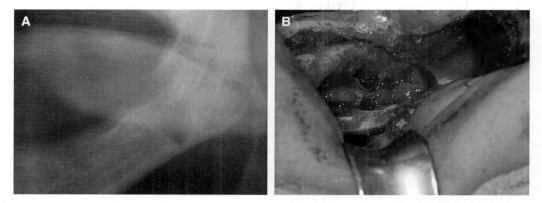

Fig. 5. (*A*) Panoramic radiograph of patient who sustained IAN injury after removal of third molar in an edentulous mandible. (*B*) Clinical photograph demonstrates microrepair of the IAN injury depicted in (*A*).

attractive alternative to grafting because there is no donor site morbidity and the alloplast theoretically could guide the regenerating axons and prevent displacement or rotation of the proximal and distal nerve stumps. Clinical results have not been consistent, however, and alloplastic materials are not generally recommended for peripheral trigeminal nerve reconstruction [25]. Vein grafting also has been described as an alternative to autogenous grafting. Clinical results demonstrated that continuity defects repaired with vein grafts for the IAN demonstrated outcomes comparable to autogenous nerve grafts when completed through an extraoral approach. Lingual nerve defects repaired with vein grafts demonstrated acceptable sensory recovery with defects smaller than 5 mm. This success may be related to the lingual nerve surgical procedure being

performed intraorally and the fact that the vein graft may collapse or kink with movements of the tongue [26]. Another alternative to autogenous nerve grafting is the use of skeletal muscle interpositional grafts [27].

Outcomes of trigeminal nerve microsurgery

The clinical literature on the microsurgical repair of trigeminal nerve injuries and their postoperative outcomes is limited, with most data derived from case reports and case series. Dodson and Kaban [28] completed an evidence-based medicine study to develop treatment guidelines based on the results described from clinical studies. Their summary recommendations for the operative management of trigeminal nerve injuries

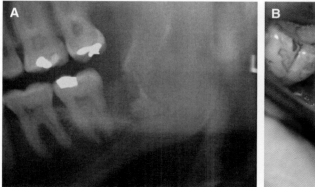
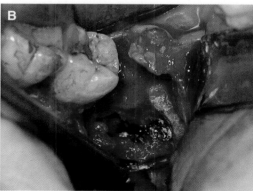

Fig. 6. (*A*) Radiograph of patient who underwent intentional partial odontectomy to avoid potential IAN injury and who continued to have persistent hypoesthesia after surgery. (*B*) Surgical view after external and internal decompression of the IAN and removal of root fragment.

include (1) tension-free primary repair whenever possible, (2) use of autogenous nerve grafts when direct primary repair is not possible, and (3) use autogenous nerve grafts or hollow conduits used for entubilization of nerve gaps 3 cm or smaller when direct repair is not possible.

Pogrel [29] reviewed his patients evaluated in a 5-year period with a diagnosis of lingual and IAN injuries. The patients who met his criteria for trigeminal nerve microsurgery were compared with patients who did not meet the criteria, and results for patients who underwent microsurgery were evaluated. In this study of 880 consecutive patients, 96 patients met the criteria for microsurgery and 51 patients had a microsurgical procedure. No differences were noted in the results based on gender, with slightly better success in the IAN group compared with the lingual nerve group. Repairs completed before 10 weeks after injury appeared to do better than late repairs, although results of neurosensory testing and patients' subjective evaluations did not always correlate. No patients developed dysesthesia postoperatively when it did not exist preoperatively. The author concluded that in select cases, trigeminal microsurgery can provide a reasonable result in improved sensation for inferior alveolar and lingual nerve injuries, with more than 50% of patients experiencing some sensory improvement.

Patients with chronic pain after trigeminal nerve injuries may have varied outcomes based on their specific presenting pain complaints. Gregg [30,31] reviewed outcomes for microsurgery in this population and found an overall reduction in pain severity of approximately 50%. The greatest reduction in pain was observed in patients diagnosed with hyperalgesia (61%) and hyperpathia (58%) compared with patients with anesthesia dolorosa and sympathetic mediated pain, who had pain reduction of approximately 15% and 21%, respectively. Patients who have central deafferentation pain pose the greatest challenge to the clinician because of lack of diagnostic or predictive tests. Treatments for central deafferentation pain generally involve use of anticonvulsant agents in combination with tricyclic antidepressants or psychotropic agents. Patients who have dysesthesia may have more psychiatric issues than patients who present with no pain [32]. It is incumbent upon the microsurgeon to rule out centrally mediated pain, which has a poor prognosis with microsurgery.

End-organ receptor regeneration has been demonstrated by Zuniga and colleagues [33] using methylene blue staining and videophotography of the fungiform papillae of the tongue. The reduction in the number of fungiform papillae, pores, and ratio of pores per papilla demonstrated that severe lingual nerve injuries resulted in a sensorineural taste disorder. The progressive increase in the number of fungiform papillae, pores, and ratio of pores per papillae along with increased response to citric acid stimuli after microsurgical repair of the lingual nerve in 50% of cases provide evidence that taste may regenerate after the lingual nerve repair. Transected lingual nerves that undergo microsurgical repair can result in the recovery of taste, regeneration of fungiform taste receptors, and recovery of some neurosensory function. Early repair of complete lingual nerve injuries is recommended to provide the optimal chance for some gustatory return [34].

Sensory re-education

Sensory re-education may help patients maximize their quality of sensory recovery. Patients must be educated preoperatively as to what can be expected realistically after trigeminal nerve microsurgery. All patients initially are anesthetic in the region of the nerve repair postoperatively. Dysesthesias are usually diminished or eliminated in this immediate period; however, usually some sensitivity is noted in the affected area. The innervated zone should be stimulated with different textures to create the varied perceived sensations. Patients could stroke the area with a cotton swab while looking in the mirror and focus on fine touch and directional sense. Alternatively, they may stimulate the area with toothbrush bristles to facilitate fine touch, pressure, and directional movements. The goal of sensory re-education is to stimulate the peripheral receptors so that the central nervous system can begin processing this information again.

Patients must understand clearly that most likely they will never experience complete sensory recovery and probably will always have some subjective feeling of altered sensation. The goal is for this sensory deficit not to interfere with activities of daily living. Some unpleasant sensations and the feelings of tingling, electrical shocks, and crawling within the affected region can occur early in the healing process. These feelings are to be expected. More complex sensory functions, such as vibration, fine touch, and directional sense, can be delayed for up to 1 year, which indicates the importance of serial examinations to demonstrate areas of improvement. The perceived changes occur so slowly that the patient has difficulty interpreting any significant improvement. After examination, it is important to discuss their improvement and review how certain abnormal behaviors, such as tongue biting, drooling, and food incompetence, have dissipated and protective reflexes have returned. The sensory levels achieved by 1 year are basically the final level obtained by patients.

Summary

Injury to peripheral branches of the trigeminal nerve, namely the lingual and inferior alveolar branches, is a known complication of third molar surgery. Surgeons should inform patients preoperatively of this risk as part of the informed consent process and closely monitor any patients postoperatively who present with hypoesthesia or dysesthesia. It is imperative that surgeons document the extent of injury and perform some basic neurosensory function testing in the postoperative period. Any patient who does not resolve spontaneously should be referred to a surgeon skilled in trigeminal nerve microsurgery for assessment and possible treatment. Trigeminal nerve microsurgery has been demonstrated to improve sensory function in these patients.

References

[1] Eliav E, Gracely RH. Sensory changes in the territory of the lingual and inferior alveolar nerves following lower third molar extraction. Pain 1998;77: 191–9.

[2] Akal UK, Sayan NB, Aydogan S, et al. Evaluation of the neurosensory deficiencies of oral and maxillofacial region following surgery. Int J Oral Maxillofac Surg 2000;29:331–6.

[3] Venta I, Lindqvist C, Ylipaavalniemi P. Malpractice claims for permanent nerve injuries related to third molar removals. Acta Odontol Scand 1998;56:193–5.

[4] Ziccardi VB, Assael LA. Mechanisms of trigeminal nerve injuries. Atlas Oral Maxillofac Surg Clin North Am 2001;9:1–11.

[5] Hill CM, Mostafa P, Thomas DW, et al. Nerve morbidity following wisdom tooth removal under local and general anaesthesia. Br J Oral Maxillofac Surg 2001;39:423–8.

[6] Brann CR, Brickley MR, Shepherd JP. Factors influencing nerve damage during lower third molar surgery. Br Dent J 1999;186:514–6.

[7] Rehman K, Webster K, Dover MS. Links between anaesthetic modality and nerve damage during lower third molar surgery. Br Dent J 2002;193:43–5.

[8] Gulicher D, Gerlach KL. Sensory impairment of the lingual and inferior alveolar nerves following removal of impacted mandibular third molars. Int J Oral Maxillofac Surg 2001;30:306–12.

[9] Behnia H, Kheradvar A, Shabrohhi M. An anatomic study of the lingual nerve in the third molar region. J Oral Maxillofac Surg 2000;58:649–51.

[10] Miloro M, Halkias LE, Slone HW, et al. Assessment of the lingual nerve in the third molar region using magnetic resonance imaging. J Oral Maxillofac Surg 1997;55:134–7.

[11] Valmaseda-Castellon E, Berini-Aytes L, Gay-Escoda C. Lingual nerve damage after third lower molar surgical extraction. Oral Surg Oral Med Oral Pathol Oral Radiol Endod 2000;90:567–73.

[12] Pichler JW, Beirne OR. Lingual flap retraction and prevention of lingual nerve damage associated with third molar surgery: a systematic review of the literature. Oral Surg Oral Med Oral Pathol Oral Radiol Endod 2001;91:395–401.

[13] Seddon HJ. Three types of nerve injury. Brain 1943; 66:237–88.

[14] Sunderland S. A classification of peripheral nerve injury producing loss of function. Brain 1951;74: 491–516.

[15] Dao TTT, Mellor A. Sensory disturbances associated with implant surgery. Int J Prosthodont 1998; 11:462–9.

[16] Zuniga JR, Meyer RA, Gregg JM, et al. The accuracy of clinical neurosensory testing for nerve injury diagnosis. J Oral Maxillofac Surg 1998;56:2–8.

[17] Zuniga JR, LaBanc JP. Advances in microsurgical nerve repair. J Oral Maxillofac Surg 1993;51(Suppl 1):62–8.

[18] Joshi A, Rood JP. External neurolysis of the lingual nerve. Int J Oral Maxillofac Surg 2002;31:40–3.

[19] Meyer RA. Applications of microneurosurgery to the repair of trigeminal nerve injuries. Oral Maxillofac Surg Clin North Am 1992;4:405–16.

[20] Terzis J, Faibisoff B, Williams HB. The nerve gap: suture under tension versus graft. Plast Reconstr Surg 1975;56:166.

[21] Eppley BL, Snyders RV. Microanatomic analysis of the trigeminal nerve and potential nerve graft donor sites. J Oral Maxillofac Surg 1991;49:612–8.

[22] Pogrel AM, Renaut A, Schmidt B, et al. The relationship of the lingual nerve to the mandibular third molar region: an anatomic study. J Oral Maxillofac Surg 1995;53:1176–81.

[23] Brammer JP, Epker BN. Anatomic-histologic survey of the sural nerve: implications for inferior alveolar nerve grafting. J Oral Maxillofac Surg 1988;46:111–7.

[24] Wolford LM. Autogenous nerve graft repairs of the trigeminal nerve. Oral Maxillofac Surg Clin North Am 1992;4:447–57.

[25] Pitta MC, Wolford LM, Mebra P, et al. Use of Gore-Tex tubing as a conduit for inferior alveolar and lingual nerve repair: experience with 6 cases. J Oral Maxillofac Surg 2001;59:493–6.

[26] Pogrel MA, Magben A. The use of autogenous vein grafts for inferior alveolar and lingual nerve reconstruction. J Oral Maxillofac Surg 2001;59:985–8.

[27] Rath EM. Skeletal muscle autograft for repair of the human inferior alveolar nerve: a case report. J Oral Maxillofac Surg 2002;60:330–4.

[28] Dodson TB, Kaban LB. Recommendations for management of trigeminal nerve defects based on a critical appraisal of the literature. J Oral Maxillofac Surg 1997;55:1380–6.

[29] Pogrel MA. The results of microneurosurgery of the inferior alveolar and lingual nerve. J Oral Maxillofac Surg 2002;60:485–9.

[30] Gregg JM. Studies of traumatic neuralgia in the maxillofacial region: symptom complexes and response to microsurgery. J Oral Maxillofac Surg 1990;48:135–40.

[31] Gregg JM. Studies of traumatic neuralgias in the maxillofacial region: surgical pathology and neural mechanisms. J Oral Maxillofac Surg 1990;48: 228–37.

[32] Sandstedt P, Sorensen S. Neurosensory disturbances of the trigeminal nerve: a long-term follow-up of traumatic injuries. J Oral Maxillofac Surg 1995;53: 498–505.

[33] Zuniga JR, Chen N, Phillips CL. Chemosensory and somatosensory regeneration after lingual nerve repairs in humans. J Oral Maxillofac Surg 1997;55: 2–13.

[34] Hillerup S, Hjorting-Hansen E, Reumert T. Repair of the lingual nerve after iatrogenic injury: a follow-up study of return of sensation and taste. J Oral Maxillofac Surg 1994;52:1028–31.

ELSEVIER
SAUNDERS

Oral Maxillofacial Surg Clin N Am 19 (2007) 117–128

ORAL AND
MAXILLOFACIAL
SURGERY CLINICS
of North America

Complications of Third Molar Surgery

Gary F. Bouloux, MD, BDS, MDSc, FRACDS, FRACDS(OMS),
Martin B. Steed, DDS, Vincent J. Perciaccante, DDS*

*Division of Oral and Maxillofacial Surgery, Emory University School of Medicine, 1365-B Clifton Road NE,
Suite 2300-B, Atlanta, GA 30322, USA*

In 1994, the American Association of Oral and Maxillofacial Surgeons Third Molar Clinical Trial research group began an ambitious longitudinal study that has added an immense amount of scientific data to our understanding of third molar surgery outcomes. Concurrently, the American Association of Oral and Maxillofacial Surgeons identified the need to characterize the clinical outcomes of procedures commonly performed by members of the specialty in the 1990s [1]. As a result, an outcomes assessment committee was created to design ways to track and evaluate the results of oral and maxillofacial surgical procedures. These procedures included the extraction of third molars—the most commonly performed procedure by oral and maxillofacial surgeons. A recent retrospective cohort study by Bui and colleagues [2] evaluated the multivariate relationships among risk factors and complications for third molar removal. These efforts represent a continued movement toward the use of evidence-based medicine to elucidate outcomes to help provide more accurate risk:benefit ratios and allow surgeons to better predict the incidence of complications and identify individuals likely to experience them.

Third molar extraction remains one of the most ubiquitous procedures performed by oral and maxillofacial surgeons, and most third molar surgeries are performed without intra- or postoperative difficulties. In all surgical procedures, proper preoperative planning and the blending of surgical technique with surgical principles is of paramount importance for decreasing the incidence of complications. Third molar removal is no different, yet such a common procedure sometimes results in what are relatively rare complications. The possibility of these events should be discussed with patients before the procedure and handled in a timely and corrective manner by the surgeon. Complications related to third molar removal range from 4.6% to 30.9% [2,3]. They may occur intraoperatively or develop in the postoperative period.

The four most common postoperative complications of third molar extraction reported in the literature are localized alveolar osteitis (AO), infection, bleeding, and paresthesia. Major complications discussed in this article, such as mandibular fracture, severe hemorrhage, or iatrogenic displacement of third molar teeth, are rare and as such, studies that evaluate incidence or predisposing factors are difficult to carry out and the literature is limited.

This article addresses the incidence of specific complications and, where possible, offers a preventive or management strategy. Injuries of the inferior alveolar and lingual nerves are significant issues that are discussed separately in this text [4]. Periodontal defects also may follow third molar surgery and are discussed elsewhere in this text [5]. Surgical removal of third molars is often associated with postoperative pain, swelling, and trismus. They are expected and typically transient and are not considered complications or discussed further.

Factors thought to influence the incidence of complications after third molar removal include age, gender, medical history, oral contraceptives, presence of pericoronitis, poor oral hygiene, smoking, type of impaction, relationship of third molar to the inferior alveolar nerve, surgical time,

---

* Corresponding author.

E-mail address: vpercia@emory.edu
(V.J. Perciaccante).

1042-3699/07/$ - see front matter © 2007 Elsevier Inc. All rights reserved.
doi:10.1016/j.coms.2006.11.013

surgical technique, surgeon experience, use of perioperative antibiotics, use of topical antiseptics, use of intra-socket medications, and anesthetic technique [1–3,6–19]. Many studies are retrospective, subject to selection bias, or poorly controlled for confounding variables, however. Conclusions drawn from individual studies are often not in agreement, which makes an evidence-based preventive or management approach challenging.

Complications that are discussed further include AO, postoperative infection, hemorrhage, oro-antral communication (OAC), damage to adjacent teeth, displaced teeth, and fractures.

Alveolar osteitis

AO is a clinical diagnosis characterized by the development of severe, throbbing pain several days after the removal of a tooth and often is accompanied by halitosis. The extraction socket is often filled with debris and is conspicuous by the partial or complete loss of the blood clot. The frequency of AO ranges from 0.3% to 26% [1–3,6,8,9,11,12,14,16]. AO is known to occur more frequently with mandibular third molar extraction sockets, although the exact reason is not clear [1,3]. The cause of AO is also poorly understood. Birn [20] suggested that AO is the result of release of tissue factors leading to the activation of plasminogen and the subsequent fibrinolysis of the blood clot. This also may explain the apparent increased incidence of AO when the surgery is more difficult and traumatic. Nitzan [21] suggested that AO is primarily the result of a localized bacterial infection. It is likely that AO is a result of a complex pathophysiology that involves a localized bacterial infection and subsequent fibrinolysis.

In an extensive review of the literature, Alexander [22] found numerous studies that supported increasing age, female gender, oral contraceptives, smoking, surgical trauma, and pericoronitis as risk factors for AO, although a significant number of studies also refuted these purported associations. The same author found a majority of studies that supported the use of generous intraoperative lavage, perioperative antiseptic mouth wash, intra-alveolar medicaments, and systemic antibiotics to reduce the incidence of AO. Unfortunately, however, the literature concerning AO is not consistent. Two recent prospective studies comparing systemic perioperative metronidazole with placebo found the incidence of AO

and early postoperative infection to be the same [7,23]. Based on these studies, metronidazole cannot be recommended for the prevention of AO, although the results cannot be extrapolated to the use of all systemic antibiotics. Despite the abundance of obligate and facultative anaerobic micro-organisms in odontogenic infections and possibly AO, it is possible that a more appropriate perioperative antimicrobial would reduce the incidence of AO. Perioperative ampicillin recently was found to reduce clinical recovery time when compared with placebo, although no specific comment was made regarding the incidence of AO or infection [24]. Postoperative antibiotics are generally not considered efficacious in reducing the incidence of AO or infection [25].

The incidence of AO after third molar removal may be reduced by adopting several approaches that, although not universally accepted, are based on the best literature currently available. First, third molars should be removed only when preexisting pericoronitis has been treated adequately. Oral hygiene also should be satisfactory before the surgical procedure. Second, the surgery should be completed as atraumatically as possible using copious irrigation when a drill/bur is needed to remove bone or section teeth. Third, an intra-alveolar antibiotic, such as tetracycline, may be beneficial when placed in the socket before closure [22,26]. The amount of antibiotic should be kept to a minimum to help reduce the likelihood of a giant cell reaction or myospheruloma formation. Finally, chlorhexidine 0.12% mouthwash should be used on the day of surgery and for several days thereafter [10].

The management of AO is less controversial than the etiology and prevention. A combination of antibacterial dressings, obtundant dressings, and topical anesthetic agents is used to alleviate severe pain. A multitude of different medicaments and carrier systems are commercially available with little scientific evidence to guide the choice. The authors have used alvogyl containing butamben, eugenol, and iodoform with good success. Eugenol is a phenolic compound that denatures protein, is neurotoxic, and interrupts neural transmission, whereas iodoform is an antibacterial agent. Patients should be seen regularly after placement of the dressing, which may need to be changed several times to eliminate the symptoms. The use of intra-alveolar dressings in sockets when the inferior alveolar neurovascular bundle is exposed is not recommended. Systemic analgesics may be used as an adjunct, but they are often unnecessary after local management measures have been undertaken.

Infections

Postoperative infections after third molar removal have been reported to vary from 0.8% to 4.2% [1–3,6,11,12,14,16]. Infections may develop in the early or late postoperative period, with mandibular third molar sites more commonly affected [1,3]. It has been suggested that age, degree of impaction, need for bone removal or tooth sectioning, exposure of the inferior alveolar neurovascular bundle, presence of gingivitis or pericoronitis, surgeon experience, use of antibiotics, and location of surgery (hospital versus office procedure) are all risk factors for postoperative infections [3,6,11–14,16]. The benefit of perioperative or postoperative systemic antibiotics on the incidence of infection remains questionable and cannot be recommended currently [7,18,23,25,27]. Perioperative antibiotics are discussed in detail elsewhere in this issue [18]. Odontogenic infections—both pre- and postoperative—are typically mixed infections with a predominance of anaerobic microorganisms, although streptococci are usually the largest single group of organisms [28,29]. When infections develop they can spread in multiple directions depending on the anatomic location of the infection and adjacent tissue planes. Maxillary third molar infections may extend to the maxillary vestibule, buccal space, deep temporal space, or infratemporal fossa. Mandibular third molar infections may spread to the mandibular vestibule, buccal space, submasseteric space, pterygomandibular space, parapharyngeal space, or submandibular space. Parapharyngeal and submandibular infections may produce significant airway embarrassment. Infections also may involve the retropharyngeal tissues and subsequently the mediastinum, with disastrous results.

The management of postoperative infection involves the systemic administration of appropriate antibiotic and surgical drainage. Penicillin continues to be a good first choice antibiotic given the mixed nature of the infection and the presence of streptococci, although increasing resistance to penicillin has been reported [29,30]. Amoxicillin may be substituted because it has a wider spectrum of activity and is only dosed two or three times a day. Metronidazole also can be added to the antibiotic regimen to increase coverage against anaerobic organisms. Penicillin or amoxicillin and metronidazole (either alone or in combination) continue to be the antimicrobials of choice in the United Kingdom [31,32]. The use of clindamycin as an alternative has become popular because it provides aerobic and anaerobic coverage [33]. The choice of antibiotic should be made carefully considering the likely micro-organisms involved, the potential for allergic reactions, side effects, and complications, such as the increased risk for the development of pseudomembranous colitis with broad-spectrum antibiotics, such as clindamycin.

Bleeding and hemorrhage

The reported range of clinically significant bleeding as a result of third molar extraction has ranged from 0.2% to 5.8% and can be classified as either intra- or postoperative with causes that can be local or systemic. In the recent American Association of Oral and Maxillofacial Surgeons Age-Related Third Molar Study, the investigators found an intraoperative frequency of unexpected hemorrhage of 0.7% and a postoperative frequency of unexpected or prolonged hemorrhage of 0.1% [1]. In a study of 583 patients, Bui and colleagues [2] found the frequency of clinically significant bleeding to be 0.6% and noted that the variability on reported rates is at least partly a result of varying definitions. This value is similar to that found by Chiapasco and colleagues [11], in which they found excessive intraoperative bleeding in 0.7% of mandibular third molars and a 0.6% incidence of postoperative excessive bleeding. Maxillary third molars showed a 0.4% incidence of postoperative excessive bleeding. A higher incidence of excessive hemorrhage was found in distoangular teeth, deep impactions, and older patients. Excessive hemorrhage resulting from extraction of mandibular molars is more common than bleeding from maxillary molars (80% and 20%, respectively) [34].

The causes of hemorrhage can be either local or systemic in nature. Systemic conditions, such as hemophilia A or B and von Willebrand's disease, are often identified early in a patient's life and extractions can be approached in a systematic manner to maximize the patient's ability to form a stable clot. Patients with severe hemophilia A who have been treated previously with plasma-derived or recombinant factor VIII products may develop inhibitors to the factor products and prove to be difficult to manage, however. Alloantibodies against foreign factor VIII develop in

25% to 30% of patients with severe hemophilia A who receive therapeutic infusions of factor VIII [35]. The inhibitor level is measured in Bethesda Units, and patients are placed into either a low or high responder group. Approximately 75% of patients fall within the high responder group. The therapy of choice for patients who have hemophilia with inhibitors is the induction of immune tolerance, and multiple protocols exist to achieve this, including the Bonn protocol and the Malmoe regimen. In the preparation for an elective procedure in a patient in whom long-term immune tolerance has not been accomplished, recombinant FVIIa (Novo-Seven) and activated prothrombin complex concentrates with FVIII inhibitor bypass activity (FEIBA) are well-established therapeutic modalities [35]. FEIBA contains the proenzymes of prothrombin complex proteins II,VII, IX, and X and small amounts of their activation products. Its effects occur mainly through factors II, Xa, and V–dependent activation of the clotting cascade and avoid dependence on factor VIII. There are difficulties with Novo-Seven and FEIBA related to difficulty in determining correct dosage and lack of laboratory tests capable of determining dosage sufficiency [35]. Management of these patients should include close coordination with a hematologist and the maximal use of local measures, including the fabrication of an individually fitted dressing plate before surgery.

Antithrombotic medications, such as Coumadin (warfarin sodium), can be discontinued if medically feasible, switched via protocol to a heparin regimen during the perioperative period, or dealt with in a local manner in an anticipatory fashion.

Local factors that result from soft-tissue and vessel injury represent the most common cause of postoperative hemorrhage and respond best to local control, which includes meticulous surgical technique with avoidance of the inferior alveolar neurovascular bundle and particular care at the distolingual aspect of the mandible. Patients who experience continued postoperative bleeding should be instructed to apply gauze pressure to the extraction site for 45 minutes. The patient's medical history should be reinvestigated and vital signs should be monitored. If the application of pressure proves unsuccessful, the patient and the extraction site should be examined closely. Local anesthesia administered at this time should not contain a vasoconstrictor to enable accurate identification of the cause of bleeding. The

extraction site may be curetted and suctioned gently. If the bleeding is from soft tissue and is arterial in nature but does not involve the neurovascular bundle, it is usually amenable to cautery. Bony bleeders may be managed with bone wax or various hemostatic agents (Table 1). These materials may be stabilized and maintained within the socket with sutures. Oral fibrinolysis from salivary enzymes may play a role in some cases, and the use of fibrin-stabilizing factors, such as epsilon-aminocaproic acid (Amicar) or tranexamic acid (Cyclokapron), may be helpful (Table 1).

Massive intraoperative bleeding is a rare occurrence and can be secondary to a mandibular arteriovenous malformation, which can be either low flow (venous) or high flow (arterial). The presence of such a malformation in the maxilla or mandible is potentially life threatening secondary to unmanageable bleeding upon attempted tooth extraction. Eight percent of patients died as a result of massive bleeding during tooth extraction in the series reported by Guibert-Tranier and colleagues [36]. Arteriovenous malformations are a rare condition in the maxillofacial region, occurring with a higher incidence in other regions of the body. Arteriovenous malformations in the maxillofacial region are often apparent on physical examination and panoramic radiography. A history of recurrent spontaneous bleeding from the gingival is the most frequent objective sign. Other physical findings include gingival discoloration, hyperthermia over the lesion, a subjective feeling of pulsation, and the presence of a palpable bruit. Mandibular arteriovenous malformations usually appear as multilocular radiolucencies on radiographic studies, although significant lesions may be nonapparent [37]. Angiography is necessary and essential to confirm the diagnosis and assess the extent and vascular architecture of the lesion [38]. Treatment of mandibular arteriovenous malformations involves either surgical excision or embolization. Multiple reports describing the use of permanent embolic agents support their use and suggest that many arteriovenous malformations whose angioarchitecture support transvenous approach can be cured without surgical resection.

Damage to adjacent teeth

The incidence of damage to adjacent restorations of the second molar has been reported to be 0.3% to 0.4% [11]. Teeth with large restorations or carious lesions are always at risk of fracture

Table 1
Local hemostatic agents useful for oral bleeding

Name	Source	Action	Application
Gelfoam	Absorbable gelatin sponge	Scaffold for blod clot formation	Place into socket and retain in place with suture
Surgicel	Oxidized regenerated methylcellulose	Binds platelets and chemically precipitates fibrin through low pH	Place into socket (Note: cannot be mixed with thrombin)
Avitene	Microfibrillar collagen	Stimulates platelet adherence and stabilizes clot; dissolves in 4–6 weeks	Mix fine powder with saline to desired consistency
Collaplug	Preshaped, highly cross-linked collagen plugs	Stimulates platelet adherence and stabilizes clot; dissolves in 4–6 weeks	Place into extraction site
Collatape	Highly crosslinked collagen	Stimulates platelet adherence and stabilizes clot; dissolves in 4–6 weeks	Place ribbon into extraction site
Thrombin	Bovine thrombin (5000 or 10,000 U)	Causes cleavage of fibrinogen to fibrin and positive feedback to coagulation cascade	Mix fine powder with $CaCl_2$ and spray into area desired; alternatively, mix with Gelfoam before application
Tiseel	Bovine thrombin, human fibrin, $CaCl_2$, and aprotinin	Antifibrinolytic action of aprotinin	Requires specialized heating, mixing and delivery system; inject into extraction site

Adapted from Moghadam H, Caminiti MF. Life threatening hemorrhage after extraction of third molars: case report and management protocol. J Can Dent Assoc 2002;68(11):671.

or damage upon elevation. Correct use of surgical elevators and bone removal can help prevent this occurrence. Discussion should take place preoperatively with patients at high risk. Maxillary mesioangular impactions with a Pell and Gregory class B (crown to cervical relationship) and mandibular vertical impactions may be at a slightly higher risk [11].

Mandibular fracture

Mandibular fracture as a result of third molar removal is a recognized complication and has important medicolegal and patient care implications. It should be included on all third molar extraction consent forms. Mandibular fracture during or after surgical third molar removal is a rare but major complication. The incidence of mandibular fracture during or after third molar removal has been reported to be 0.0049% [39].

Other studies cite even lower incidence. Alling and colleagues [40] retrospectively showed an intraoperative mandibular fracture rate of 1 in 30,583 patients and a postoperative rate of 1 in 23,714, whereas Nyul [41] reported one fracture in 29,000 cases.

Possible predisposing conditions, such as increased age, mandibular atrophy, the concurrent presence of a cyst or tumor, and osteoporosis, have been implicated in increasing the risk of mandible fracture. The preangular region of the mandible is an area of lowered resistance to fracture secondary to its thin cross-sectional dimension, and an impacted tooth occupies a relatively significant space within the bone of this region. The concurrent presence of a dentigerous or follicular cyst around the third molar or a radicular cyst around the second molar and removal of the tooth and any surrounding bone necessary to mobilize it further mechanically weakens this area. Studies that have attempted to characterize the small number of patients who have experienced a mandibular fracture after or during extraction of a third molar include Iizuka and colleagues [42], who retrospectively evaluated the clinical and radiographic data of 12 patients with 13 mandible fractures after removal of wisdom teeth. They found that patients older than 30 to 40 years with tooth roots superimposed on the inferior alveolar canal or adjacent to the canal on panoramic evaluation are at increased risk for fracture. The study found few intraoperative fractures (one) and found that the late fractures (eight) occurred on average 6.6 days after the surgery exclusively upon mastication. Libersa and colleagues [39] evaluated 37 fractures from 750,000 extractions and identified 17 intraoperative fractures and 10 late fractures. Of the 10 late fractures, 8 occurred in men and 6 occurred during mastication. Most late fractures occurred between 13 and 21 days after surgery, which could be caused by an increase in masticatory function and occlusal forces outstripping the bony healing.

Exclusively late fractures were found in a study by Krimmel and Reinert [43] in a retrospective series of six patients who sustained mandibular fracture from third molar removal. The fractures occurred 5 to 28 days (mean, 14 days) after the tooth removal. The ages of all six patients were between 42 and 50 and all had full dentition. Pell and Gregory vertical classifications for the teeth were Class B in two cases and Class C in four cases. The authors concluded that the major risk factor for the complication seemed to be advanced age in combination with a full dentition.

Regardless of the mechanism, mandibular fractures that occur during or soon after the extraction of a mandibular third molar are usually nondisplaced or minimally displaced. Such hairline fractures that extend from an extraction site are not always easily identified, and clinical suspicion may require CT if the initial panoramic film produces negative results. The practitioner should treat the fracture definitively just as if the patient were a trauma patient. Failure to do so may result in further complications.

Maxillary tuberosity fracture

Fracture of the maxillary tuberosity on extraction of maxillary third molars is a clinically known occurrence. The anatomic position at the end of the dentoalveolar arch is such that the

posterior portion has no support, and the internal composition may be significantly maxillary sinus or soft osteoporotic bone. Preoperative radiographic evaluation of the sinus proximity and bone thickness can help anticipate tuberosity fracture. In a study by Chiapasco and colleagues [11], the extraction of 500 maxillary impacted third molars was accompanied by three fractures of the maxillary tuberosity, indicating an incidence of 0.6%. Two instances occurred with teeth classified as class C (crown to root position) by the Pell and Gregory classification scheme, whereas one was class B (crown to cervical position). The fractures occurred with equal incidence in all patient age groups.

Upon encountering a fractured tuberosity during an erupted third molar extraction, the surgeon must revisit the reason why the tooth was to be extracted in the first place. If the tooth is asymptomatic, it may be left in place and the region stabilized with an arch bar. If the tooth is infected or symptomatic and the extraction must be completed, then the tuberosity can be separated from the tooth with a high-speed hand piece and the roots sectioned. The tooth can be removed atraumatically and the tuberosity assessed for viability through evaluation of the attached periosteum and vascular supply. Attention must be given to fastidious closure of palatal and buccal mucosal tears. Possible preventive measures include use of a periosteal elevator to ensure separation of the periodontal ligament from the tooth and palpation with a finger from the nonoperating hand to evaluate the expansion of the cortical plate upon luxation.

Displacement of third molars

Maxillary third molars

Iatrogenic displacement of maxillary third molars can occur, although it is a rarely reported complication with an unknown incidence. Maxillary third molars that are superiorly positioned may have only a thin layer of bone posteriorly separating them from the infratemporal space. The tooth can be displaced in a posterosuperior direction into the infratemporal space if distal elevation is not accompanied by a retractor placed behind the tuberosity within the designed mucoperiosteal flap (Fig. 1). The literature shows that management of a third molar displaced into the infratemporal space is varied. Venous bleeding from the pterygoid plexus often makes intraoral

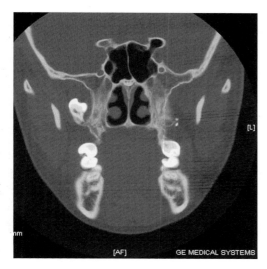

Fig. 1. Coronal cut CT. Bony window of a maxillary third molar #01 displaced into the right infratemporal fossa.

visualization of the tooth difficult [44]. Observation may be chosen but can require secondary removal in the setting of infection, limited range of motion, or a patient's wishes to have the tooth removed. Delayed removal after fibrosis takes place around the tooth also has been advocated because it can more readily be localized radiographically and intraoperatively. This secondary procedure is often completed in the operating room under general anesthesia after a CT scan is obtained to precisely locate the tooth position. Various approaches to retrieving a tooth in the infratemporal space have been described, including an intraoral approach from a sagittal split osteotomy incision, a hemicoronal approach, and manipulating the tooth via a straight needle placed cutaneously in an inferior direction and delivering it through an intraoral incision [45].

Displacement of a maxillary third molar into the maxillary sinus also can occur and has been reported [46–48]. Excessive apical force and incorrect surgical technique are thought to be the most common cause. The accepted treatment of such a displaced tooth is removal to prevent future infections. Pogrel [44] stated that the initial attempt at retrieval should be a suction placed at the opening into the sinus. If suction applied to the opening does not allow delivery, then the sinus may be irrigated with saline and the suction tip reapplied to the opening. If the second attempt is unsuccessful, further attempts should be stopped and the

patient placed on a course of antibiotics and nasal decongestants. Retrieval can be accomplished with a Caldwell-Luc approach at a second procedure in concert with closure of the oro-antral fistula and an intranasal antrostomy to facilitate maxillary sinus drainage [44].

There seems to be some discussion as to the timing of this removal. Sverzut and colleagues [48] stated that the removal should be accomplished during the same procedure but indicated that delayed treatment does not always precipitate active sinus disease and that this asymptomatic interval can last several months.

Mandibular third molars

Mandibular third molars can be iatrogenically displaced into the sublingual, submandibular, pterygomandibular, and lateral pharyngeal spaces [46,49–51]. Anatomic considerations, such as a distolingual angulation of the tooth, thin or dehisced lingual cortical plate, and excessive or uncontrolled force upon luxation, are important factors that can lead to this complication.

Lower third molars that are pushed through a perforation in the thin lingual alveolar bone normally pass inferiorly to the mylohyoid muscle. Pogrel [44] recommended that the operator place his or her thumb underneath the inferior border of the mandible in an attempt to direct the tooth back along the lingual surface of the mandible. The lingual gingiva may be reflected as far as the premolar region and the mylohyoid muscle incised to gain access to the submandibular space and deliver the tooth. In this approach, care should be taken to avoid injury to the lingual nerve in this anatomic region. Locating the displaced tooth is challenging secondary to limited working area and hemorrhage with resultant compromised visualization and blind probing that may result in further displacement. Yeh [46] described a technique that is a combination intraoral and lateral neck approach in which the original wound is extended lingually to the distal of the first molar. A 4-mm skin incision is made in the submandibular region and a hemostat inserted along the lingual surface of the mandible to stabilize the tooth while the surgeon palpates the tooth with an index finger. A Kelly clamp can be inserted to deliver the tooth upward into the mouth. The author believed this approach prevents further displacement of the tooth and limits the length of lingual flap reflection necessary.

Gay-Escoda and colleagues [51] reported a case in which a patient underwent unsuccessful extraction of a displaced mandibular third molar that was found between the platysma and sterno-cleidomastoid muscle. It was removed via a trans-cutaneous approach and the authors stated that the tooth may have undergone progressive exteriorization as a result of a prolonged inflammatory reaction.

Esen and colleagues [50] described a case in which a patient presented months after attempted extraction of a mandibular third molar with progressive limitation in mouth opening, left neck edema, and difficulty swallowing. A panoramic film was obtained and revealed a tooth in the pterygomandibular region. CT scans showed the precise location of the tooth at the anterior border of the lateral pharyngeal space underlying the left tonsillar region. The tooth was removed transorally from the tonsillar fossa (after completion of a tonsillectomy) through a vertical incision from the tonsillar fossa to the retromolar trigone.

Delayed intervention in the setting of a displaced tooth into the lateral pharyngeal space carries the risk of infection, thrombosis of the internal jugular vein, erosion of the carotid artery or one of its branches, and interference with cranial nerves IX through XII [50].

Displaced roots

Maxillary and mandibular root tips rarely may be displaced into the aforementioned spaces. The management of these displaced roots remains much the same. A mandibular third molar root may be displaced into the inferior alveolar canal. Attempts at retrieval may further injure the neurovascular bundle and should be limited to one attempt with suction.

Aspiration

All third molar extraction procedures carry the risk of tooth aspiration. The use of properly placed oropharyngeal gauze is essential in preventing this complication. The use of intravenous deep sedation by definition compromises the protective reflexes of the airway. The aspiration or swallowing of a tooth or portion of a tooth is usually the result of a patient coughing or gagging.

Oro-antral communication/fistula

An OAC is any opening between the maxillary sinus and the oral cavity. Without diagnosis and treatment this communication may epithelialize and become an oro-antral fistula (OAF).

OAC occurs most frequently from extraction of first molar teeth, followed by second molar teeth [52]. An incidence of 0.008% to 0.25% OAC has been reported with maxillary third molar removal [11,53]. It is likely that the incidence of OAC from maxillary third molar removal is underestimated, because it may be self-limiting in some cases and, in the case of impacted third molars, usually a flap is closed over the extraction site, leading to healing. OAC smaller than 2 mm in diameter likely closes spontaneously without any treatment [54,55].

Various methods for closure of OAC and OAF have been described over the years, including gold foil, buccal flaps, various palatal flaps, tongue flaps, pedicled buccal fat pad (PBFP), cheek flaps, and placement of bioabsorbable root analogs [56–69]. The authors prefer the use of the PBFP for closure of OAFs.

The buccal fat pad was first described by Heister in 1732 as a glandular structure and recharacterized as fatty tissue by Bichat in 1802 [70]. It is a biconvex mass of fatty tissue in a fine capsule with a body and four projections; the total volume is described as approximately 10 mL [68,70–73]. The four projections are buccal, pterygoid, and superficial and deep temporal extensions. The blood supply to the buccal fat pad comes from the buccal and deep temporal branches of the maxillary, transverse facial branch of the superficial temporal, and branches of the facial arteries. The use of the PBFP for closure of OAF was first described by Egyedi in 1977 [74]. The description of this technique included the placement of a split-thickness skin graft over the PBFP. Research has shown that this graft does not need to be covered and epithelializes within a few weeks [55,70,75–77]. The procedure's reported success rate ranges from 92.8% to several reports of 100% [55,78–82].

Technique

The procedure can be performed under local anesthesia or intravenous sedation (Fig. 2). If a fistula is present, an incision with a 3-mm margin is made around the OAF. The fistula is excised or closed and inverted with a purse string suture of 3-0 chromic gut. Two divergent cuts are made from the remaining OAC extending anteriorly and posteriorly into the vestibule. The trapezoidal buccal mucoperiosteal flap is reflected. A 1-cm

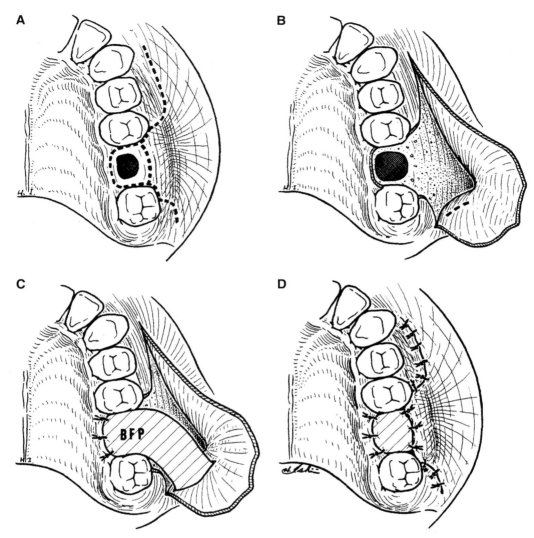

Fig. 2. The BFP method for the closure of OAF. (*A*) Incision line (*dotted line*). (*B*) The mucoperiosteal flap and the incision of the periosteum at the zygomatic buttress (*dotted line*). (*C*) Advancement of BFP into the bony defect and suturing to the palatal gingiva. (*D*) Replacement and suturing of mucoperiosteal flap into its original position. (*From* Hanazawa Y, Itoh K, Mabashi T, et al. Closure of oroantral communications using a pedicled buccal fat pad graft. J Oral Maxillofac Surg 1995;53:771; with permission. © Copyright 1995 – The American Association of Oral and Maxillofacial Surgeons.)

incision is made in the periosteum posterior to the zygomatic buttress. Curved hemostats are used to spread within the submucosal space until the fat herniates. The buccal fat pad is teased from its bed and gently advanced, without tension, and sutured to the palatal mucosa using 4-0 monofilament poliglecaprone (Monocryl) sutures. The sutures to the palate can be interrupted or, after elevation of the edge of the palatal tissue, vertical mattress sutures can be used to "tuck" the tip of

the PBFP under the edge of the palatal mucosa. The buccal flap is returned to its original position. The releasing incisions are closed and a suture is placed from the tip of the buccal flap to the PBFP, leaving the PBFP exposed to the oral cavity over the OAC. The fat epithelializes over the next few weeks. Alternatively the buccal mucoperiosteal flap may be advanced over the PBFP and primarily sutured to the palatal mucosa to form a double layered closure. Appropriate antibiotic coverage for sinus micro-organisms and decongestants are provided for 1 week. Standard sinus precautions are followed. The authors have not yet had a failure with this technique, even in smokers, although smoking cessation is strongly encouraged.

Temporomandibular joint complications

A causal relationship between the extraction of third molars and temporomandibular injury currently has little support in the literature. It has been suggested that because the procedure of extracting mandibular third molars involves the patient opening his or her mouth wide for an extended period of time and exerting a variable amount of force on the mandible, it is possible to overload or injure one or both temporomandibular joints [83]. This result would be the case especially if the surgeon did not use correct surgical technique or failed to support the mandible while removing the mandibular third molars or if the patient's protective mechanism for opening was exceeded while under general anesthesia.

In a matched case control study by Threlfall and colleagues [84], they compared 220 patients diagnosed with disc displacement with reduction to 1100 controls drawn from the participants in the 1998 UK Adult Dental Health Survey. They found that patients with diagnosed anterior disk displacement with reduction were not significantly more likely to have undergone extraction of third molars than the controls (odds ratio 1.28; confidence interval 95%). The study showed that 21 (9.5%) of the 220 patients reported that they had a third molar extracted in the 5 years before the diagnosis of an anterior disc displacement with reduction. The data did not exclude the possibility that patients who have extractions under general anesthesia and patients who have lengthy/traumatic procedures may be at increased risk of developing a temporomandibular disorder, but data did suggest that in most patients with anterior disk displacement with reduction, extraction of a third molar was unlikely to have been the etiologic factor.

Oral and maxillofacial surgeons should include an examination of the temporomandibular region, including an evaluation of joint sounds, opening and excursive movements, and temporal/masseter/pterygoid muscle tenderness in all preoperative third molar extraction patients. Care should be taken in judicious application of force and a bite block should be used to stabilize the mandible upon surgical mobilization of the lower third molar teeth.

References

[1] Haug RH, Perrott DH, Gonzalez ML, et al. The American Association of Oral and Maxillofacial Surgeons age-related third molar study. J Oral Maxillofac Surg 2005;63:1106.

[2] Bui CH, Seldin EB, Dodson TB. Types, frequencies, and risk factors for complications after third molar extraction. J Oral Maxillofac Surg 2003;61:1379.

[3] Sisk AL, Hammer WB, Shelton DW, et al. Complications following removal of impacted third molars: the role of the experience of the surgeon. J Oral Maxillofac Surg 1986;44:855.

[4] Ziccardi V, Zuniga J. Nerve injuries after third molar removal. Oral Maxillofac Surg Clin North Am 2007;19:105–15.

[5] Dodson TB. Risk of periodontal defects after third molar surgery: an exercise in evidence-based clinical decision-making. Oral Maxillofac Surg Clin North Am 2007;19:93–8.

[6] Benediktsdottir IS, Wenzel A, Petersen JK, et al. Mandibular third molar removal: risk indicators for extended operation time, postoperative pain, and complications. Oral Surg Oral Med Oral Pathol Oral Radiol Endod 2004;97:438.

[7] Bergdahl M, Hedstrom L. Metronidazole for the prevention of dry socket after removal of partially impacted mandibular third molar: a randomised controlled trial. Br J Oral Maxillofac Surg 2004;42:555.

[8] Bloomer CR. Alveolar osteitis prevention by immediate placement of medicated packing. Oral Surg Oral Med Oral Pathol Oral Radiol Endod 2000;90:282.

[9] Bruce RA, Frederickson GC, Small GS. Age of patients and morbidity associated with mandibular third molar surgery. J Am Dent Assoc 1980;101:240.

[10] Caso A, Hung L-K, Beirne OR. Prevention of alveolar osteitis with chlorhexidine: a meta-analytic review [see comment]. Oral Surg Oral Med Oral Pathol Oral Radiol Endod 2005;99:155.

[11] Chiapasco M, De Cicco L, Marrone G. Side effects and complications associated with third molar surgery. Oral Surg Oral Med Oral Pathol 1993;76:412.

[12] de Boer MP, Raghoebar GM, Stegenga B, et al. Complications after mandibular third molar extraction. Quintessence Int 1995;26:779.

[13] Figueiredo R, Valmaseda-Castellon E, Berini-Aytes L, et al. Incidence and clinical features of delayed-onset infections after extraction of lower third molars. Oral Surg Oral Med Oral Pathol Oral Radiol Endod 2005;99:265.

[14] Goldberg MH, Nemarich AN, Marco WP II. Complications after mandibular third molar surgery: a statistical analysis of 500 consecutive procedures in private practice. J Am Dent Assoc 1985;111:277.

[15] Larsen PE. Alveolar osteitis after surgical removal of impacted mandibular third molars: identification

of the patient at risk. Oral Surg Oral Med Oral Pathol 1992;73:393.

[16] Osborn TP, Frederickson G Jr, Small IA, et al. A prospective study of complications related to mandibular third molar surgery. J Oral Maxillofac Surg 1985;43:767.

[17] Pogrel MA. Complications of third molar surgery. In: Kaban LB, Pogrel MA, Perrot DH, editors. Complications of oral and maxillofacial surgery. Philadelphia: WB Saunders Co.; 1997. p. 59–68.

[18] Mehrabi M, Allen JM, Roser SM. Therapeutic agents in perioperative third molar surgical procedures. Oral Maxillofac Surg Clin North Am 2007; 19:69–84.

[19] Susarla S, Blaeser B, Magalnick D. Third molar surgery and associated complications. Oral Maxillofac Surg Clin North Am 2003;15:177.

[20] Birn H. Etiology and pathogenesis of fibrinolytic alveolitis. Int J Oral Surg 1973;2:211.

[21] Nitzan DW. On the genesis of "dry socket." J Oral Maxillofac Surg 1983;41:706.

[22] Alexander RE. Dental extraction wound management: a case against medicating postextraction sockets. J Oral Maxillofac Surg 2000;58:538.

[23] Sekhar CH, Narayanan V, Baig MF. Role of antimicrobials in third molar surgery: prospective, double blind, randomized, placebo-controlled clinical study. Br J Oral Maxillofac Surg 2001;39:134.

[24] Foy SP, Shugars DA, Phillips C, et al. The impact of intravenous antibiotics on health-related quality of life outcomes and clinical recovery after third molar surgery. J Oral Maxillofac Surg 2004;62:15.

[25] Poeschl PW, Eckel D, Poeschl E. Postoperative prophylactic antibiotic treatment in third molar surgery: a necessity? [see comment]. J Oral Maxillofac Surg 2004;62:3.

[26] Blum IR. Contemporary views on dry socket (alveolar osteitis): a clinical appraisal of standardization, aetiopathogenesis and management: a critical review [see comment]. Int J Oral Maxillofac Surg 2002;31:309.

[27] Bulut E, Bulut S, Etikan I, et al. The value of routine antibiotic prophylaxis in mandibular third molar surgery: acute-phase protein levels as indicators of infection. J Oral Sci 2001;43:117.

[28] Peltroche-Llacsahuanga H, Reichhart E, Schmitt W, et al. Investigation of infectious organisms causing pericoronitis of the mandibular third molar. J Oral Maxillofac Surg 2000;58:611.

[29] Quayle AA, Russell C, Hearn B. Organisms isolated from severe odontogenic soft tissue infections: their sensitivities to cefotetan and seven other antibiotics, and implications for therapy and prophylaxis. Br J Oral Maxillofac Surg 1987;25:34.

[30] Labriola JD, Mascaro J, Alpert B. The microbiologic flora of orofacial abscesses. J Oral Maxillofac Surg 1983;41:711.

[31] Falconer DT, Roberts EE. Report of an audit into third molar exodontia. Br J Oral Maxillofac Surg 1992;30:183.

[32] Gill Y, Scully C. The microbiology and management of acute dentoalveolar abscess: views of British oral and maxillofacial surgeons. Br J Oral Maxillofac Surg 1988;26:452.

[33] Kirkwood KL. Update on antibiotics used to treat orofacial infections. Alpha Omegan 2003;96:28.

[34] Jensen S. Hemorrhage after oral surgery: an analysis of 103 cases. Oral Surg Oral Med Oral Pathol 1974; 37:2.

[35] Heiland M, Weber M, Schmelzle R. Life-threatening bleeding after dental extraction in a hemophilia A patient with inhibitors to factor VIII: a case report received from University Hospital Hamburg-Eppendorf, Hamburg, Germany. J Oral Maxillofac Surg 2003;61:1350.

[36] Guibert-Tranier F, Piton J, Riche MC, et al. Vascular malformations of the mandible (intraosseous haemangiomas): the importance of preoperative embolization. A study of 9 cases. Eur J Radiol 1982; 2:257.

[37] Larsen PE, Peterson LJ. A systematic approach to management of high-flow vascular malformations of the mandible. J Oral Maxillofac Surg 1993;51:62.

[38] Kawano K, Mizuki H, Mori H, et al. Mandibular arteriovenous malformation treated by transvenous coil embolization: a long-term follow-up with special reference to bone regeneration. J Oral Maxillofac Surg 2001;59:326.

[39] Libersa P, Roze D, Cachart T, et al. Immediate and late mandibular fractures after third molar removal. J Oral Maxillofac Surg 2002;60:163.

[40] Alling C, Alling R. Indications for management of impacted teeth. In: Alling C, Helfrick J, Alling R, editors. Impacted teeth. Philadelphia: WB Saunders Co.; 1993. p. 43–64.

[41] Nyul L. Kieferfracturen bei zahnextractionen. Zahlärztl Welt 1959;60.

[42] Iizuka T, Tanner S, Berthold H. Mandibular fractures following third molar extraction: a retrospective clinical and radiological study. Int J Oral Maxillofac Surg 1997;26:338.

[43] Krimmel M, Reinert S. Mandibular fracture after third molar removal. J Oral Maxillofac Surg 2000; 58:1110.

[44] Pogrel M. Complications of third molar surgery. Oral Maxillofac Surg Clin North Am 1990;2:441.

[45] Gulbrandsen SR, Jackson IT, Turlington EG. Recovery of a maxillary third molar from the infratemporal space via a hemicoronal approach. J Oral Maxillofac Surg 1987;45:279.

[46] Yeh C-J. A simple retrieval technique for accidentally displaced mandibular third molars. J Oral Maxillofac Surg 2002;60:836.

[47] Patel M, Down K. Accidental displacement of impacted maxillary third molars. Br Dent J 1994;177:57.

[48] Sverzut CE, Trivellato AE, Lopes LM dF, et al. Accidental displacement of impacted maxillary third molar: a case report. Braz Dent J 2005;16:167.

[49] Ertas U, Yaruz MS, Tozoglu S. Accidental third molar displacement into the lateral pharyngeal space. J Oral Maxillofac Surg 2002;60:1217.

[50] Esen E, Aydogan LB, Akcali MC. Accidental displacement of an impacted mandibular third molar into the lateral pharyngeal space. J Oral Maxillofac Surg 2000;58:96.

[51] Gay-Escoda C, Berini-Aytes L, Pinera-Penalva M. Accidental displacement of a lower third molar: report of a case in the lateral cervical position. Oral Surg Oral Med Oral Pathol 1993;76:159.

[52] Ehrl PA. Oroantral communication: epicritical study of 175 patients, with special concern to secondary operative closure. Int J Oral Surg 1980;9:351.

[53] Punwutikorn J, Waikakul A, Pairuchvej V. Clinically significant oroantral communications: a study of incidence and site. Int J Oral Maxillofac Surg 1994;23:19.

[54] Schuchardt K. Treatment of oro-antral perforations and fistulae. Int Dent J 1955;5.

[55] Hanazawa Y, Itoh K, Mabashi T, et al. Closure of oroantral communications using a pedicled buccal fat pad graft. J Oral Maxillofac Surg 1995;53:771.

[56] Sachs SA, Kay SA, Specter J, et al. Treatment of a persistent oro-antral fistula with a posteriorly based lateral tongue flap. Int J Oral Surg 1979;8:225.

[57] Carstens MH, Stofman GM, Sotereanos GC, et al. A new approach for repair of oro-antral-nasal fistulae: the anteriorly based buccinator myomucosal island flap. J Craniomaxillofac Surg 1991;19:64.

[58] Yamazaki Y, Yamaoka M, Hirayama M, et al. The submucosal island flap in the closure of oro-antral fistula. Br J Oral Maxillofac Surg 1985;23:259.

[59] Berger A. Oroantral openings and their surgical correction. Arch Otolaryngol 1939;30:400.

[60] Goldman EH, Stratigos GT, Arthur AL. Treatment of oroantral fistula by gold foil closure: report of case. J Oral Surg (Chic) 1969;27:875.

[61] Mainous EG, Hammer DD. Surgical closure of oroantral fistula using the gold foil technique. J Oral Surg (Chic) 1974;32:528.

[62] Magnus WW, Castner DV Jr. Closure of oronasal fistula with gold plate implant. Oral Surg Oral Med Oral Pathol 1971;31:460.

[63] Fredrics HJ, Scopp IW, Gerstman E, et al. Closure of oroantral fistula with gold plate: report of case. J Oral Surg (Chic) 1965;23:650.

[64] Killey HC, Kay LW. An analysis of 250 cases of oroantral fistula treated by the buccal flap operation. Oral Surg Oral Med Oral Pathol 1967;24:726.

[65] James RB. Surgical closure of large oroantral fistulas using a palatal island flap. J Oral Surg (Chic) 1980;38:591.

[66] Ito T, Hara H. A new technique for closure of the oroantral fistula. J Oral Surg (Chic) 1980;38:509.

[67] Thoma K, Pajarola GF, Gratz KW, et al. Bioabsorbable root analogue for closure of oroantral communications after tooth extraction: a prospective case-cohort study. Oral Surg Oral Med Oral Pathol Oral Radiol Endod 2006;101:558.

[68] Cheung LK, Samman N, Tideman H. Reconstructive options for maxillary defects. Ann R Australas Coll Dent Surg 1994;12:244.

[69] Awang MN. Closure of oroantral fistula. Int J Oral Maxillofac Surg 1988;17:110.

[70] Tideman H, Bosanquet A, Scott J. Use of the buccal fat pad as a pedicled graft. J Oral Maxillofac Surg 1986;44:435.

[71] Dubin B, Jackson IT, Halim A, et al. Anatomy of the buccal fat pad and its clinical significance. Plast Reconstr Surg 1989;83:257.

[72] Stuzin JM, Wagstrom L, Kawamoto HK, et al. The anatomy and clinical applications of the buccal fat pad [see comment]. Plast Reconstr Surg 1990; 85:29.

[73] Tostevin PM, Ellis H. The buccal pad of fat: a review. Clin Anat 1995;8:403.

[74] Egyedi P. Utilization of the buccal fat pad for closure of oro-antral and/or oro-nasal communications. J Maxillofac Surg 1977;5:241.

[75] Stajcic Z, Todorovic L, Pesic V, et al. Tissucol, gold plate, the buccal fat pad and the submucosal palatal island flap in closure of ororantral communication. Dtsch Zahnarztl Z 1988;43:1332.

[76] Loh FC, Loh HS. Use of the buccal fat pad for correction of intraoral defects: report of cases. J Oral Maxillofac Surg 1991;49:413.

[77] Hai HK. Repair of palatal defects with unlined buccal fat pad grafts. Oral Surg Oral Med Oral Pathol 1988;65:523.

[78] Abuabara A, Cortez ALV, Passeri LA, et al. Evaluation of different treatments for oroantral/oronasal communications: experience of 112 cases. Int J Oral Maxillofac Surg 2006;35:155.

[79] Stajcic Z. The buccal fat pad in the closure of oroantral communications: a study of 56 cases. J Craniomaxillofac Surg 1992;20:193.

[80] Baumann A, Ewers R. Application of the buccal fat pad in oral reconstruction. J Oral Maxillofac Surg 2000;58:389.

[81] Martin-Granizo R, Naval L, Costas A, et al. Use of buccal fat pad to repair intraoral defects: review of 30 cases. Br J Oral Maxillofac Surg 1997;35:81.

[82] Dolanmaz D, Tuz H, Bayraktar S, et al. Use of pedicled buccal fat pad in the closure of oroantral communication: analysis of 75 cases. Quintessence Int 2004;35:241.

[83] Huang GJ, LeResche L, Critchlow CW, et al. Risk factors for diagnostic subgroups of painful temporomandibular disorders (TMD). J Dent Res 2002;81:284.

[84] Threlfall AG, Kanaa MD, Davies SJ, et al. Possible link between extraction of wisdom teeth and temporomandibular disc displacement with reduction: matched case control study. Br J Oral Maxillofac Surg 2005;43:13.

Oral Maxillofacial Surg Clin N Am 19 (2007) 129–136

ORAL AND
MAXILLOFACIAL
SURGERY CLINICS
of North America

Legal Implications of Third Molar Removal

James R. Hupp, DMD, MD, JD, MBA

Department of Oral and Maxillofacial Surgery, School of Dentistry,
University of Mississippi Medical Center, 2500 North State Street, Jackson, MS 39216-4505, USA

The exposure and removal of impacted teeth is a challenging task. The varying shapes and root patterns, proximity to significant blood vessels, nerves, sinuses and adjacent teeth, differing degrees and angles of impaction, and limitations on a patient's ability to open or otherwise cooperate during a procedure near the rear of the mouth results in an infinite number of clinical presentations facing the surgeon. It is not surprising that undesired outcomes can and do occur, even under the best of circumstances and surgical execution.

When less than ideal results occur after a clinical procedure, a chance of legal action by the patient arises. This occurrence is even more likely when the patient did not have serious preoperative symptoms, as is the case in many patients having impacted teeth managed. The risk of a lawsuit also rises during management of impacted teeth because of the regular intravenous administration of potent anesthetic agents.

Fortunately, the surgical treatment of impactions has a low complication rate [1–3]. Surgeons who perform surgery for thousands of impactions each year run only a small risk of being sued. Even when everything done for a patient falls within the standards of good medical/dental care, however, a patient may resort to litigation if he or she decides or is convinced by someone that an injury resulted because of doctor error.

This article focuses on legal ramifications inherent in the management of impacted teeth. The initial section explores the potential problems associated with the care of impacted teeth that makes such treatment clinically challenging and legally risky. The next section discusses means of preventing or mitigating the injuries that can occur during or after impaction surgery. The final sections cover various strategies to consider should a problem occur or legal action seem imminent.

Legal exposure associated with third molars

The malpractice carrier that covers the greatest number of oral and maxillofacial surgeons in the United States recently had the percentages of malpractice claims shown in Table 1. The high number of lawsuits initiated because of nerve injury and removal of the wrong tooth is not surprising—not so much because of their relatively high percentages, but because of the level of concern such outcomes cause the affected patients.

Injury to branches of the trigeminal nerve during lower third molar surgery are remarkably rare considering how anatomically close the impacted teeth and the surgery needed to treat them are to major nerve trunks [4]. The roots of fully formed impacted lower third molars are often less than 2 mm from the inferior alveolar nerve (IAN) canal and regularly are directly on or beside the canal [5]. In rare cases, IAN canals run between the roots of lower third molars or are even surrounded by the roots (Fig. 1).

The lingual nerve commonly runs against or close to the lingual cortex of the mandible in the area of lower third molars. It also can run along or even over the rest the bone distal to the second or third molar [1,6,7]. The lingual and IAN are also put at risk due to where local mandibular anesthetic blocks are delivered near the lingula [8,9].

Although an exhaustive review of the pathophysiology of nerve injury is beyond the scope of this article, a quick review of various types of nerve injury is useful [10,11]. The most common form of peripheral nerve injury related to surgery

E-mail address: jhupp@sod.umsmed.edu

Table 1
Relative incidence of legal actions based on problems related to dental surgery

Problem	% of Claims
Nerve damage	14
Wrong tooth removed	14
Poor result	9
Infection	7
Improper surgery	7
Injury adjacent to surgical site	4
Failure to properly diagnose	3
Surgical complication	2.5
Retained foreign body	2.5
Temporomandibular joint problems	2
Others	35

(*Data courtesy of* OMS National Insurance Co., Rosemont, IL)

is caused by compression or excess stretching of a nerve. This condition can cause neurapraxia, in which the axon and nerve sheath maintain continuity but normal nerve function is disrupted. During surgery to remove impacted lower third molars, stretching most commonly affects the lingual nerve when the surgeon attempts to have it retracted out of the way to provide exposure of the surgical field and protect the nerve and soft tissue from sharp instruments or rotary equipment. The lingual nerve is susceptible in many cases when it lays in intimate contact with bone just lingual to an impacted tooth. Because most surgeons do not attempt to widely expose the lingual bone, the nerve is "tented up" by the retractor and risks injury. Studies have shown an increase in lingual nerve injuries when surgeons attempt to use a retractor to protect the nerve during surgery for third molars [1,12–14]. Compression of nerves during impaction surgery is believed to occur most often when a tooth with root laying close to the IAN canal is rotated in a manner that pivots the root into the canal and causes compression of the nerve by the canal wall, by the root itself, or both.

The next more severe form of nerve injury, axonotmesis, involves disruption of the axon while the neural sheath maintains its continuity. This type of damage typically results from excessive stretching of the nerve trunk. The most likely site for this injury is where the lingual nerve comes in close relationship with the site of lower third molar impaction surgery. As for as neurapraxia, prevention involves eliminating or limiting the retraction of soft tissue lingual to the third molar operative site.

Clearly the worst form of nerve injury is partial or complete severance of the nerve trunk, which can occur because of incisions, elevation of flaps, curettage of the socket after surgery when a nerve has been exposed, or cutting of the nerve by drill burs or chisels [1]. The IAN and lingual nerve are at risk of this form of injury. Prevention of this kind of injury is discussed later in this Article.

There are three other means by which the IAN and lingual nerve are vulnerable to injury. Rotary instruments cause a large amount of frictional heat when being used to remove bone or divide a tooth. If insufficient cooling irrigation is not delivered to the point of heat generation, it is conceivable that such heat could radiate to nearby nerves and cause thermal damage. Similarly, caustic chemicals or agents with highly unphysiologic pH could cause

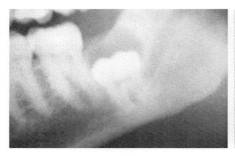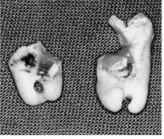

Fig. 1. Radiographic view of mandibular third molar suggests that it is surrounding or adjacent to inferior alveolar canal (*left*). Hole and indentation in roots of mandibular third molar indicates position of roots in relation to the inferior alveolar canal. When this tooth was removed the inferior alveolar neurovascular bundle was severed (*right*). (Note that the radiograph is not of this tooth). (*From* Peterson LJ, Ellis E III, Hupp JR, et al, editors. Contemporary oral and maxillofacial surgery. 4th edition. St. Louis (MO): Mosby; 2003. p. 200.)

chemical damage to nerves if the substance comes in contact with the nerve. Finally, the lingual nerve runs a highly variable course. In some cases the nerve runs close to or in the soft tissue covering the occlusal surface of the impaction socket. If a suture is placed too far lingually, it could incorporate the nerve in the suture as it is tied, compressing the nerve and causing it to malfunction [1].

The second most common reason for malpractice suits against oral and maxillofacial surgeons is removal of the wrong tooth. Although this occurrence is less likely with third molars than other teeth in the mouth, it occasionally occurs when other molar teeth are missing or in unusual positions. More likely than removal of the wrong tooth during impaction surgery is injury to an adjacent tooth or soft tissue. Many impactions are difficult to approach, causing the surgeon sometimes to exert pressures that may affect the second molar. If the second molar has a large distal amalgam or a crown, the restoration can be dislodged or damaged. Problems also can occur if rotary instruments inadvertently come in contact with the second molar. Soft tissue is also at risk from rotary and sharp instruments. The lips, tongue, and buccal mucosa can be damaged by being cut or burned while the surgeon is conducting impaction surgery.

Fortunately, complete fracture of the jaw is rare during impaction removal procedures. Fractures of substantial portions of the maxillary tuberosity can occur when removing impacted upper third molars, however. Mandibular fractures can occur when a person has an unusually weak jaw because of disease, the lower third molar and its socket or associated pathology (ie, cyst) make up a large percentage of the cross-sectional diameter of the mandible, when an impacted lower third molar thins the cortical bone of the inferior border of the mandible, when a chisel is used on a previously elevated tooth, when excessive force is used during elevation, or a chisel is used to remove a lower third molar [1,15].

Infections after impaction removal are surprisingly rare in healthy patients, although surgery is done in a "dirty" field. Infection occurs primarily because of the extremely rich vascular supply of the oral and maxillofacial region. Infections do occur even when proper perioperative procedures are followed, however [15]. Fortunately, these infections rarely cause serious problems if diagnosed and promptly addressed.

Severe hemorrhage after third molar surgery is another unusual occurrence. Typically, such bleeding indicates a coagulopathy or unusual pathology or anomalies in the wound bed.

Displacement of all or part of a third molar into the sinus or other spaces is uncommon. Displacement most often occurs during impaction surgery when an upper third molar enters the pterygoid space posterior to the tuberosity. Root tips can enter the maxillary sinus or be dislodged into sublingual space through the lingual cortical plate adjacent to impacted lower teeth. A serious type of displacement occurs when an extracted tooth or tooth part falls into a patient's oropharynx. From there it can be aspirated easily into the larynx or lungs or be swallowed. A tooth entering the gastrointestinal tract is unlikely to cause anything more than some temporary emotional problems for a patient, whereas aspiration can lead to partial or complete airway obstruction or laryngospasm. If a tooth reaches the bronchi or lungs, even if a serious obstruction does not occur, the tooth still represents a nidus for infection and requires bronchoscopic removal.

Impacted maxillary third molars are usually directly in contact with the wall of the maxillary sinus; however, sinus communications with the oral cavity through the surgical site rarely occur or become symptomatic.

Occasionally, it becomes necessary to electively abandon the effort to remove all parts of an impacted tooth. This decision is wise when further surgery would place either a nerve or the maxillary sinus in jeopardy. Sometimes parts of an impacted tooth are accidentally left behind because of problems with visibility or when the tooth was partially ankylosed. Foreign bodies, such as amalgam from another tooth, also can be left in an extraction socket, particularly if a lower socket is exposed while work is done on maxillary teeth. Broken bur bits or broken needle pieces also can find their way into extraction sockets.

Removal of lower third molars can put considerable forces on the mandible and the temporomandibular joint, particularly if steps are not taken to sufficiently divide a tooth or remove bone. If the surgeon or an assistant does not provide counterpressure or a stabilizing pressure on the mandible, damage to the temporomandibular joint can occur and result in pain or other forms of dysfunction.

Two final issues associated with impaction surgery that can lead to legal problems relate to nonsurgical aspects of care. The first is the process of informed consent, in which a patient gives a care provider permission to "touch his/her body." In American and other societies, people are not allowed to intentionally touch another person without that person's consent. To touch someone without his or her agreement is considered assault and battery. For surgeons, the informed consent process has evolved to a point at which the standard of care expects patients to be informed of what procedure is planned, the significant risks of that procedure, reasonable alternatives to the procedure, and who is performing the procedure. Although most people focus on the informed consent form, the process of reasonably informing a patient usually requires more, such as verbal discussions, diagrams, brochures, or informative videos. Failure to get proper informed consent from a patient before impaction surgery can leave a surgeon in legal difficulty even if the surgery proceeds without incident or complications.

The other nonsurgical legal problem a surgeon who performs impaction surgery can face is failure to adequately document the surgical and anesthetic aspects of the procedure. When no complications happen, this is unlikely to bother the surgeon legally (although third party reimbursement may be jeopardized). If a patient suffers postoperative problems, however, the surgeon may find it difficult to mount a successful legal case to defend himself or herself if important aspects of the patient's care were not documented, including follow-up visits and other communications.

Lessening risks associated with impaction surgery

Although many undesired outcomes after third molar impaction surgery are unavoidable, some steps can be taken before and during surgery to control the risk or help mitigate any damages. This begins at the time of diagnosis and treatment planning [16,17]. Certain factors that increase the chance of complications can be determined as the surgeon analyzes the case preoperatively. Studies have shown that the incidence of IAN damage rises above age 25 to 30 [2,18–20], which may mean that patients older than 25 or 30 should only have impacted lower third molars removed if there are signs or symptoms of associated pathologic condition. Perhaps these patients should have only the coronal portion of the third molar removed if surgery is indicated [18].

The presence of acute infection at the site of an impacted tooth is known to increase the incidence of postoperative infection. If an acute or subacute infection is present, the surgeon might treat the soft tissue infection with antibiotics and irrigation to get resolution before impaction surgery. This approach also lowers the frequency of postoperative osteitis sicca, lessens bleeding during and after surgery, and improves the healing potential of the soft tissues.

Removal of the wrong tooth is less common in third molar surgery than for other dental extractions. Caution is still necessary to ensure that the referring doctor's wishes are followed and that a tooth is not misidentified during surgery. Referral slips with diagrams on which the teeth planned for removal care are clearly marked are a good way to minimize communication errors. Surgeons also should perform their own evaluations of which teeth require removal to ensure it coincides with the referring doctor's plans. If there is any confusion, a surgeon should contact the referring provider to clarify the situation. Finally, the author suggests that while removing third molars the surgeon audibly count the first and second molars before beginning to elevate a third molar.

The degree and angulation of an impacted third molar and the proximity to the IAN, adjacent teeth, and maxillary sinus should guide the planned surgical procedure. Any images obtained of teeth planned for removal should show the entire tooth to be extracted and important nearby structures. If they do not, additional views should be obtained. Images also should be up-to-date. If radiographs or visual inspection indicates that the restoration of a tooth adjacent to the impaction is at risk during surgery, this information should be told to the patient.

Investigators have found that certain patterns of the radiographic relationship between the roots of impacted teeth and the IAN are associated with a higher likelihood of IAN injury [2,20–23]:

- Darkening of tooth root at the inferior alveolar canal
- Narrowing of tooth root at the inferior alveolar canal
- Interruption of "white lines" (cortical bone) of the inferior alveolar canal adjacent to tooth apices
- Diversion of inferior alveolar canal when adjacent to tooth apices
- Highly hooked roots near inferior alveolar canal

When such patterns are present, it may be wise to forego removal of that tooth or do a coronal resection only.

Once treatment planning is complete, the surgeon can proceed to informing the patient of recommendations, material risks, and reasonable alternatives*, which can be done with a combination of written and visual materials and a discussion between the surgeon and the patient (or parent or guardian when applicable). The person responsible for giving consent also should be allowed to ask questions.

In the end, if a case goes to trial the jury is asked to determine if a risk would have been material to them before agreeing to the procedure. This decision is usually balanced against the potential emotional damage done to a patient if a surgeon would list every possible risk, no matter how trivial or rare.

The final aspect of the informed consent process is the informed consent document, which should include the planned procedure, surgeon and others given permission to carry out the procedure, material risks, sensible alternatives, and a statement that the consenting adult had the opportunity to ask questions before signing the form. Forms should be customized sufficiently so only risks and alternatives that apply to the procedure being performed on the patient are included. The document should have a place for signature of a witness who was present while risks and alternatives were being presented (preferably someone other than the doctor or relative of the patient).

Once the surgeon is ready to proceed with impaction surgery there are steps to take to lessen the chance of some of the complications discussed previously. This section does not provide a detailed description of how to remove impacted third molars, however.

As in all open surgery, the principle of having good visibility is important when removing buried teeth. Good lighting, effective suctioning, and sufficient access via mouth-opening devices (eg, bite-blocks) and reflection of soft tissue flaps are all important. The reflection of soft tissue to gain access usually involves a scalpel incision. The most critical aspect of making incisions for third molar surgery from a legal risk standpoint is to avoid coming near the lingual nerve. Because this nerve can run at or even lateral to the crest of the lingual bone lingual to the retromolar pad, it is best to make any incision in this area well to the buccal aspect of this area. In most cases this means keeping the incision over the crest of the buccal cortical plate as it runs toward the ascending ramus [1].

Reflection of soft tissue is typically uncomplicated, but surgeons should use great care when deciding if or how much to reflect on the lingual aspect of lower third molars [1,24,25]. In most cases impacted lower teeth can be removed successfully with minimal lingual soft tissue retraction.

When bone removal or tooth division is necessary to remove an impacted tooth, most surgeons use high-speed, high-torque rotary drills. The heat that these drills create can cause damage at the operative site or to other oral tissues against which the shaft of the bur or the motor of the handpiece rests. If access is inadequate to avoid causing thermal damage to adjacent soft tissues, greater access should be gained or a nonconductive barrier, such as a thick wet gauze, should be placed between the handpiece and the soft tissue. Heat at the site of surgery is usually effectively contained by high volumes of irrigating fluid delivered right at the point where the bur engages hard tissues.

While using a drill to remove bone or divide a tooth, care is required to avoid damage to an adjacent tooth, the IAN canal, or the lingual nerve. For avoidance of nerve injury the surgeon must remain vigilant of coming close to the nerves with the bur, which often necessitates keeping the bur within tooth structure as one approaches the lingual side of the tooth. With respect to the IAN and the maxillary sinus, this may require stopping drill use once the crown of an impacted third molar is removed if the preoperative assessment of the patient shows the sinus or IAN in close proximity to the apices.

When elevating impacted teeth it is important to avoid excessive forces, because it may fracture the bone, dislodge an adjacent tooth or its restoration, or rotate the root of a lower tooth into the IAN canal. In most circumstances the need to use increased force to elevate a tooth signals the need for division of the tooth, the need for bone removal, or creation of a purchase point in the impacted tooth.

---

* "Material risks" is a legal concept in which the frequency of a risk is balanced against the severity of damage the risk entails. Relatively common risks that cause only minor damage might be mentioned, such as excessive bleeding, whereas rare risks that can cause significant problems for a patient, such as nerve injury, also should be mentioned. Similarly, although a life-threatening reaction to a drug used during surgery is rare, it also should be mentioned in writing because of the obviously catastrophic impact on the patient. Conversely, it can be debated whether possibility of jaw fracture merits mention because it is rare and the long-term consequences to the patient are relatively minor.

Sometimes after good efforts are made to remove an impacted tooth entirely, portions of the roots still remain, possibly because of partial ankylosis, extreme curvature of the apices, or other factors. If these apices are near the IAN or maxillary sinus it may be wise to abandon efforts to remove them because the risks of removal may be higher than risks of leaving them behind. The patient should be alerted to this decision so proper follow-up can be arranged.

Once all or most of an impacted tooth is removed, any points of elevation against bone should be smoothed with a bone file and copious irrigation under pressure should be used to rinse the wound free of debris and lower the bacterial count. When a residual follicle remains in the extraction socket or soft tissue hemorrhage is problematic, the surgeon should use care when grasping tissue on the lingual aspect of the wound. The lingual nerve may be inadvertently engaged and damaged. While closing the wound of lower third molar sites, the surgeon should take care to take a limited bite of lingual tissue to avoid impaling the lingual nerve with the needle or encircling the nerve in the suture [26].

The patient or escort should be given detailed postoperative instructions. It is beneficial for someone to review these directions verbally with the patient or escort to ensure that there are no questions. It is good practice to include in instructions the way to contact the doctor or covering doctor should problems or questions arise after the patient leaves. Many surgeons use the effective practice and risk management technique of calling the patient the evening after surgery to check that all is well.

Actions should complications occur

The management of complications associated with third molar impaction surgery is beyond the scope of this article; however, some general guidelines of what to do should a complication occur may help lower legal exposure. As in most aspects of life, people prefer to be told of problems when they occur rather than discover them on their own later from another practitioner. This is true of delays or cancellations in the airline industry, government mix-ups, and surgical problems. If the surgeon notes a complication during or after surgery, he or she should immediately alert the patient or guardian, explain its implications, and discuss ways to mitigate any damages.

In most circumstances the surgeon should not admit error immediately because in most cases an error did not occur or the suspected error may not actually have caused the problem. Similarly, the decision to not bill the patient when a complication occurs is unsound in most situations, because this fact might be construed later as an admission of responsibility for causing the complication. The author believes it is unwise, however, to send such patients' bills to a collection agency should they not pay for the procedure.

If a surgeon is fully capable of managing the complication, he or she should proceed to do so, while keeping careful records of everything done and said to the patient. If the complication is one that the surgeon is not completely prepared to manage, however, he or she should enlist the help of another practitioner. For instance, if a nerve injury occurs and the surgeon does not commonly handle such problems, referral to another person trained to manage nerve injuries should be made, particularly once it is clear the nerve is not rapidly recovering [27]. Similarly, if an infection fails to respond to the usual measures that typically resolve the problem, assistance from another health care provider may be useful.

Careful written documentation of the complication and all steps taken to lessen any damages is important. Care should be taken when deciding if and how to photo-document any problems, however. Most malpractice liability insurance carriers require policy holders to notify them if an event occurs that creates significant legal exposure. For problems that arise from care provided in a hospital or surgery center, risk management units often expect to be alerted when serious complications happen. In that case the risk managers can be helpful in working with the doctor and patient to minimize the chance of legal action.

Actions if legal action is imminent

Direct or indirect evidence of a lawsuit after a problem related to impaction surgery should trigger certain actions by the doctor. Direct evidence might be receipt of a subpoena for a patient's records or delivery of a complaint by an attorney. Indirect evidence includes requests for records by the patient or attorney or comments referencing plans for legal action made by a patient or family or friends. In either case the doctor should immediately secure all records related to that patient, including imaging, billing records, information about appointments made or missed, prescriptions given to the patient, and records of any phone, normal mail, or e-mail communications with the patient or about the patient with other health care providers. The consent form and evidence of any brochures or other items given to the patient also should be kept in a place to which only the doctor has access. This approach makes certain nothing is lost, tampered with, or photocopied without the doctor's consent.

The doctor's or corporation's liability carrier should be notified, even if only indirect evidence of a lawsuit exists. If a lawsuit is filed it is usually helpful to work with the liability carrier when selecting a defense lawyer, because companies sometimes do not possess enough information of who has the skills and experience necessary in a surgeon's area to handle the case. Once a legal team is identified, one should work closely with the attorney to help select credible experts to review the case and provide testimony on one's behalf. The surgeon also may consider attending the depositions the attorney conducts because the surgeon may be able to alert the attorney to questions to ask to better support the case. Some plaintiff experts also may find it more difficult to distort the truth when facing the doctor against whom they are testifying.

Once a patient initiates a lawsuit, the surgeon's relationship with him or her should change in most circumstances. The surgeon should not abandon the patient but may suggest that further care be provided by another doctor because instituting a liability suit indicates that the patient no longer fully trusts the surgeon's capabilities. The surgeon also should not discuss the suit with the patient or family or friends. If the patient's lawyers try to speak to the surgeon or staff, they should be immediately directed to your attorney.

Summary

Although complications during or after the surgical removal of impacted third molars are rare, legal exposure does arise. Fortunately, most patients understand that most complications are not caused by doctor error and do not pursue a legal course of action. There are steps to take before, during, and after surgery to lessen the chances of complications, however. If complications do arise, most can be managed without triggering the need for any involvement by the legal system.

References

[1] Merrill RG. Prevention, treatment and prognosis for nerve injury related to the difficult impaction. Dent Clin North Am 1979;23(3):471–88.

[2] Valmaseda-Castellon E, Berini-Aytes L, Gay-Escoda C. Inferior alveolar nerve damage after lower third molar surgical extraction: a prospective study of 1117 surgical extractions. Oral Surg Oral Med Oral Pathol 2001;92(4):377–83.

[3] Renton T, McGurk M. Evaluation of factors predictive of lingual nerve injury in third molar surgery. Br J Oral Maxillofac Surg 2001;39(6):423–8.

[4] Carmichael FA, McGowan DA. Incidence of nerve damage following third molar removal: a West of Scotland Oral Surgery Research Group study. Br J Oral Maxillofac Surg 1992;30:78–82.

[5] Susarla SM, Blaeser BF, Magalnick D. Third molar surgery and associated complications. Oral Maxillofacial Surg Clin North Am 2003;15:177–86.

[6] Gregg JM. Surgical management of lingual nerve injuries. Oral Maxillofac Surg Clin North Am 1992; 4(2):417–24.

[7] Kiesselback JE, Chamberlain JG. Clinical and anatomic observations on the relationship of the lingual nerve to the mandibular third molar region. J Oral Maxillofac Surg 1984;42:565–7.

[8] Pogrel MA, Thamby S. Permanent nerve involvement resulting from inferior alveolar nerve blocks. J Am Dent Assoc 2000;131(10):901–7.

[9] Pogrel MA, Schmidt BL, Sambajon V, et al. Lingual nerve damage due to inferior alveolar nerve blocks: a possible explanation. J Am Dent Assoc 2003; 134(2):195–9.

[10] La Banc JP. Classification of nerve injuries. Oral Maxillofac Surg Clin North Am 1992;4(2):285–96.

[11] Hupp JR. Management of injuries to the facial and trigeminal nerves. J Maryland Dent Assoc 1994;40: 25–9.

[12] Brahams D. Retractor design and the lingual nerve. Lancet 1992;339:801.

[13] Mason DA. Lingual nerve damage following lower third molar surgery. Int J Oral Maxillofac Surg 1988;17:290–4.

[14] Pogrel MA, Goldman KE. Lingual flap retraction for third molar removal. J Oral Maxillofac Surg 2004;62(9):1125–30.

[15] Kunkel M, Morbach T, Kleis W, et al. Third molar complications requiring hospitalization. Oral Surg Oral Med Oral Pathol Oral Radiol Endod 2006; 102(3):300–6.

[16] Caissie R, Goulet J, Fortin M, et al. Iatrogenic paresthesia in the third division of the trigeminal nerve: 12 years of clinical experience. J Can Dent Assoc 2005;71(3):185–90.

[17] Venta I, Lindqvist C, Ylipaavalniemi P. Malpractice claims for permanent nerve injuries related to third molar removals. Acta Odontol Scand 1998;56(4): 193–6.

[18] Pogrel MA, Lee JS, Muff DF. Coronectomy: a technique to protect the inferior alveolar nerve. J Oral Maxillofac Surg 2004;62(12):1447–52.

[19] Adeyemo WL. Do pathologies associated with impacted lower third molars justify prophylactic removal? A critical review of the literature. Oral Surg Oral Med Oral Pathol Oral Radiol Endod 2006;102(4):448–52.

[20] Gulicher D, Gerlach KL. Sensory impairment of the lingual and inferior alveolar nerves following removal of impacted mandibular third molars. Int J Oral Maxillofac Surg 2001;30(4):306–12.

[21] Rood JP, Nooraldeen Shehab AA. The radiological prediction of inferior alveolar nerve injury during third molar surgery. Br J Oral Maxillofac Surg 1990;28:20–5.

[22] Monaco G, Monteverchi M, Bonetti GA, et al. Reliability of panoramic radiography in evaluating the topographic relationship between the mandibular canal and impacted third molars. J Am Dent Assoc 2004;135:312–7.

[23] Albert DG, Gomes ACA, Vasconcelos RC, et al. Comparison of orthopantomographs and conventional tomography images for assessing the relationship between impacted lower third molars and the mandibular canal. J Oral Maxillofac Surg 2006; 64(7):1030–7.

[24] Pichler JW, Beirne OR. Lingual flap retraction and prevention of lingual nerve damage associated with third molar surgery: a systematic review of the literature. Oral Surg Oral Med Oral Pathol 2001;91(4): 395–401.

[25] Robinson PP, Loescher AR, Smith KG. The effect of surgical technique on lingual nerve damage during lower 3rd molar removal by dental students. Eur J Dent Educ 1999;3(2):52–5.

[26] Goldberg MH. Frequency of trigeminal nerve injuries following third molar removal [letter]. J Oral Maxillofac Surg 2005;63(12):1783.

[27] Zicarrdi VB, Assael LA. Mechanisms of trigeminal nerve injuries. Atlas Oral Maxillofac Surg Clin North Am 2001;9(2):1–11.

ELSEVIER
SAUNDERS

Oral Maxillofacial Surg Clin N Am 19 (2007) 137–140

ORAL AND
MAXILLOFACIAL
SURGERY CLINICS
of North America

Index

Note: Page numbers of article titles are in **boldface** type.

1042-3699/07/$ - see front matter © 2007 Elsevier Inc. All rights reserved.
doi:10.1016/S1042-3699(06)00121-X

oralmaxsurgery.theclinics.com